[

N
i
I
l
ı
]

g task but
stigations.
ance, this
plores the
nce on the

lgorithmic

including
Iatlab;
:e analysis;
er tracking

enting data;

clear guid-
invaluable
ort perform-
ods course.

'erformance
University,
ice Analysis
of Sport, editor of the *International Journal of Performance Analysis of Sport* and editor of the book series *Routledge ⁀⁀ Sport Performance Analysis.*

**Lucy Holmes** is Lecturer in Perfc ⁀⁀me Director for the MSc Performance An⁀ ⁀rt, Cardiff Metropolitan University, UK. ⁀⁀nce Analyst for Hockey Wales.

# Routledge Studies in Sports Performance Analysis

Series Editor
Peter O'Donoghue
*Cardiff Metropolitan University*

*Routledge Studies in Sports Performance Analysis* is designed to support students, lecturers and practitioners in all areas of this important and rapidly developing discipline. Books in the series are written by leading international experts in sports performance analysis and cover topics including match analysis, analysis of individual sports and team sports, technique analysis, data analytics, performance analysis for high performance management, and various methodological areas. Drawing on the very latest research, and introducing key concepts and best practice, the series meets a need for accessible, up-to-date texts at all levels of study and work in performance analysis.

Available in this series:

**An Introduction to Performance Analysis of Sport**
*Peter O'Donoghue*

**Data Analysis in Sport**
*Peter O'Donoghue and Lucy Holmes*

# DATA ANALYSIS IN SPORT

**PETER O'DONOGHUE AND LUCY HOLMES**

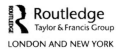

LONDON AND NEW YORK

First published 2015
by Routledge
2 Park Square, Milton Park, Abingdon, Oxon OX14 4RN

and by Routledge
711 Third Avenue, New York, NY 10017

*Routledge is an imprint of the Taylor & Francis Group, an informa business*

© 2015 Peter O'Donoghue and Lucy Holmes

*British Library Cataloguing-in-Publication Data*
A catalogue record for this book is available from the British Library

*Library of Congress Cataloging-in-Publication Data*
O'Donoghue, Peter.
Data analysis in sport / Peter O'Donoghue, Lucy Holmes.
pages cm. — (Routledge studies in sports performance analysis)
Includes bibliographical references and index.
1. Sports—Physiological aspects. 2. Sports sciences—Statistical methods.
3. Sports sciences—Research—Methodology. 4. Performance—Statistical
methods. 5. Performance—Research—Methodology. I. Holmes, Lucy
(Teacher in performance analysis) II. Title.
RC1235.O357 2015
613.7072'7—dc23
2014017975

ISBN: 978-0-415-73983-2 (hbk)
ISBN: 978-0-415-73984-9 (pbk)
ISBN: 978-1-315-81635-7 (ebk)

Typeset in Melior and Univers
by FiSH Books Ltd, Enfield

**To our parents**

# CONTENTS

# LIST OF FIGURES

# LIST OF TABLES

xii

# PREFACE

This second book in the *Routledge Studies in Sports Performance Analysis* series deals with data analysis in sports performance analysis. There are many existing textbooks on quantitative analysis, qualitative analysis and mixed methods in sport as well as more generally. The rationale for this book was that sports performance data present some unique challenges for data analysis that cannot expect to be covered by more general data analysis books. The book covers reasonably advanced material but does not go into the more advanced areas of data analytics that will be covered in a separate book within the series. The book will be of interest to performance analysts with the ambition to undertake data analysis tasks that go beyond the standard data analyses outputs provided by commercial match analysis packages. Such analysts could be working with elite athletes or in educational environments. There is a specialist modelling, profiling and statistics module within the MSc Sport Performance Analysis at the authors' university that is supported by the book. The book also serves as a reference text and, therefore, the chapters cover different aspects of data analysis rather than forming a strict sequence of chapters that must be read in order from beginning to end. The intended readership is expected to be performance analysts who are already capable of developing and using performance analysis systems. A pre-requisite to using the current textbook is that the analysts are competent users of commercial match analysis packages and are capable of developing and using sports specific systems within these packages. They should be capable of using the standard outputs of commercial packages including event lists, frequency tables of events, interactive video review facilities and highlight movie creation. There is an alternative type of reader who does not engage in system development or operation but who may be tasked with performing sophisticated analyses of sports performance data gathered by others.

Existing textbooks in sports performance analysis cover some of the standard analysis tasks performed in the area. For example, the *Routledge Handbook of Sports Performance Analysis* (McGarry *et al.*, 2013) covers profiling and reviews work done using artificial neural networks. *Research Methods in Sports Performance Analysis* (O'Donoghue, 2010) is aimed at students undertaking research projects within the final year of their undergraduate degree or masters programme and covers qualitative methods, non-parametric statistical tests and analysis of reliability that are relevant to sports performance research. *Notational Analysis of Sport* (Hughes and Franks, 2004a) contains chapters on reliability, profiling and modelling. *The Essentials of Performance Analysis of Sport* (Hughes and Franks, 2008) contains chapters on probabilistic modelling in sport and reliability. However, there are data analysis techniques that are done by performance analysts that are not covered in any textbooks. Furthermore, there are data pre-processing tasks that are necessary before many sports performance data can be analysed for reliability, and other pre-processing tasks performed on some data prior to applying statistical analyses. The current book fills some of these gaps but the authors would not claim that the book covers all of the advanced data analysis techniques that could be applied to sports performance data. For example, there is a chapter on Matlab. Matlab is a data analysis and modelling package about which several volumes of user guides have been written. Similarly, an analyst with the ability to use 10 per cent of the functionality of Microsoft Excel will be very valuable to the athletes they work with.

The book contains nine chapters, the first two of which are a natural start to the book. There was a choice of ordering of the remaining chapters, which cover different types of analysis. The first chapter discusses the nature of data and information and some general principles of data analysis. The second chapter discusses the standard data analysis features of commercial video analysis packages that readers are already expected to be familiar with. The reason for including this chapter is that many readers may use one particular package without being aware of facilities or different ways of abstracting behaviour that are used within alternative packages.

Microsoft Excel is a widely used data analysis package that many students and analysts have installed on the computers that they use. The general purpose nature of Microsoft Excel means that it can be used for more types of analyses than the analysis functions provided by commercial match analysis packages. The commercial match analysis packages provide the most fundamental analysis features for tagged video analysis. However, they cannot be expected to include all possible analysis functions for all possible sports it could be used for. This requires analysts to export data to other packages for more specialist analysis. The reason why a general purpose data analysis package like Microsoft Excel can be used is that it is such a popular package: Microsoft has been able to include wide-ranging features for statistical analysis, text processing, mathematical functions and graphics. Event lists can be exported from commercial match analysis packages and summarised using pivot tables and other functions of Microsoft Excel.

Once you have collected your data, you need to be able to present this information in a usable format for the intended viewer. Dashboards have been used in business intelligence for many years; the transfer of this knowledge to sport with the growth of the data collected was inevitable. Being able to communicate quickly and efficiently to your players, coaches and other personnel the information you have collected is vital. This presentation then becomes the first access point that allows further investigation using the performance analysis packages.

The higher-end versions of the Sportscode package provide a Statistical Window which currently has no equivalent in the alternative packages. The Statistical Window is a grid of cells that contain scripts that are programmed to calculate and display information. The scripts access data from the timeline and the information computed can be sent to the code window or an output window. There are many Sportscode users who do not use Statistical Windows within their systems. Script programming requires similar skills to other types of computer programming. A minority of skilled analysts are capable of developing systems that include Statistical Windows. The fifth chapter of the book is aimed at aspiring analysts who wish to develop this ability. It is an introduction that takes readers through three examples ranging from simple percentage calculation to a more complex example of automatically updating the score of a tennis match. Those interested in script programming should support the reading of this chapter by developing scripts of use to their own systems. Those with an ability to programme scripts can potentially work as consultants developing systems for use by other analysts working with athletes and squads.

Chapter 6 discusses the analysis of player tracking data in team sports. A variety of player tracking systems is used, ranging from relatively low-cost GPS systems to high-cost image processing systems that are used in professional soccer clubs. The player tracking systems do have analysis facilities that provide useful outputs. However, there are tactical behaviours of teams that could potentially be recognised from player tracking data. Chapter 6 proposes a five stage process of developing such algorithms using challenging in soccer as an example. Algorithms that recognise tactical aspects of collective behaviour in team sports are potentially beneficial to squads. The efficiency of an automated process allows for feedback about such behaviours to be made using quantitative information or relevant video sequences.

Matlab is a programming language and environment used for data analysis, modelling and simulation. It allows complex data structures to be created and analysed. Matlab has great potential for the analysis of sports performance data. Chapter 7 uses an example of analysing player tracking data to automatically identify where defences apply pressure, backup and cover according to Olsen's (1981) principles. A second example is a simulation system for the 2014 FIFA World Cup. There are toolkits for artificial neural networks, image processing and other advanced analyses that the book does not go into. The chapter gives readers an introduction that will allow them to start developing programming skills in Matlab. Scientific research into sports performance particularly can benefit from the use of Matlab.

Chapter 8 covers statistical analysis of sports performance data. This is a topic covered in other textbooks. However, the pre-processing of sports performance data prior to statistical analysis is of particular interest to the chapter. Many students are more than capable of selecting the correct statistical procedure to use and use statistical packages to produce statistical results. However, they sometimes have difficulty transforming data into a form that can be analysed using statistics packages. Chapter 8 discusses the use of pivot tables and other types of pre-processing that transform data into a form where they can be entered into SPSS for statistical analysis.

The final chapter covers reliability assessment in sports performance analysis. This is another area that has been covered in depth elsewhere.

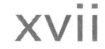

However, as with statistical analysis, data need to be transformed into a form that allows reliability statistics to be calculated. The chapter shows how timelines and event lists from independent observations can be combined to allow reliability statistics to be determined. The reliability of both input data and output information can be evaluated. An example of this is reliability assessment for commercial match analysis packages in soccer. Another issue covered in the chapter is the reliability of match statistics provided on official tournament websites.

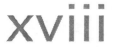

# ACKNOWLEDGEMENTS

We'd like to thank the commercial organisations who granted permission for us to use screenshots of different parts of their systems. The SPSS company granted permission to include SPSS outputs in the current book. Microsoft granted permission to use screenshots of popup windows of their system that have been used. Prozone granted permission for us to reanalyse some data used in a 2006 reliability study so that additional reliability statistics could be reported. Dartfish granted permission for us to show screenshots of different parts of the Dartfish package.

We'd also like to thank William Bailey, Josh Wells and Simon Whitmore from Routledge for their assistance during the planning and developing of this book.

Thank you all.

# CHAPTER 1

## PRINCIPLES OF DATA ANALYSIS

### INTRODUCTION

Input data are processed to produce summary output information used for decision making in practical contexts as well as to produce conclusions in academic research. Variables are used to represent different aspects of sports performance and data are measured at different levels with some header information for matches of interest being recorded before individual event records are gathered containing event details such as event type, team and player performing the event, location of the event, outcome of the event and time at which the event was performed. There are many types of data analysis including statistical analysis processes ranging from elementary descriptive and inferential statistics to multivariate predictive modelling methods. Data structures can be processed by algorithms developed in Visual BASIC or other programming languages. The most important stage of data handling is the initial determining the question being answered by the analysis. This is the purpose of the analysis and it guides both data gathering and analysis processes. There are principles of data processing that should be adhered to during any data analysis task. Davidson (1996) discussed 30 principles of data handling, 25 of which are relevant to sports performance analysis. These 25 principles and how they apply in sports performance analysis are described in this introductory chapter.

## DATA AND INFORMATION

### Abstraction and scales of measurement

All data and information are ultimately representations used for the purpose of communication (O'Donoghue, 2012: 4). Consider the simple sum 10 + 15 = 25. This could be used to represent the adding of distances, areas, times, mass, decimalised money or many other concepts measured on interval scales. Abstracting reality to numerical representations allows arithmetic to be applied to reason about situations. Abstraction is used to represent the important information of interest excluding unimportant detail not required for understanding or decision making. A simple count of passes that a player has made in a team game is information about a player's involvement in the game. This avoids going into detail about mechanical aspects of passing that may not be required to gain a sufficient understanding of the player's involvement. Equations are a form of abstraction: for example, equation (1.1) can be used to represent the percentage of passes that are successful in terms of successful passes made and total passes made. This means that we do not need to express the percentages for all possible combinations of successful pass frequencies and total pass frequencies. We can simply use equation (1.1) to represent the percentage of passes that are successful in general.

$$\text{Percentage of successful passes} = 100 \times \text{Successful passes} / \text{Total passes} \tag{1.1}$$

Not all data used in decision making are numerical as categorical variables measured on nominal or ordinal scales can also be used. An example of a nominal variable is gender, which is used to classify people into two different groups. Ordinal variables classify people or events into different categories that do have an order. For example, if we were classifying possessions in a game of soccer by outcome, some outcomes are more desirable than others. For example, we may have five outcome classes; scoring, shot on target, shot off target, entering the attacking third or not entering the attacking third. We will assume these are mutually exclusive with shots on target not including goals and possessions classified as entering the attacking third and not entering the attacking third being restricted to those not involving a scoring opportunity. Scoring is a more desirable outcome than a shot on target, which is a more desirable outcome than a shot off target, and so on. Hence this is an ordinal

2

variable. There are many different types of data (Anderson *et al.*, 1994: 8; Diamantopoulos and Schlegelmilch, 1997: 4–7) including facts, knowledge, intentions, attitudes, motives, primary and secondary data and published statistics. In sports performance analysis, categorical and numerical facts and figures are used together with more complex video information.

Scales of measurement are interesting in sports performance analysis because there is a fifth scale of measurement that is not always considered in other areas (O'Donoghue, 2010: 164–5). The four commonly known scales of measurement are nominal, ordinal, interval and ratio scales. In sports performance analysis we have variables representing different locations of the playing area; for example, a soccer pitch could be divided into 18 areas (Hughes and Franks, 2004b). The 18 areas that Hughes and Franks (2004b) denoted 'A' to 'V' are not merely different values of an ordinal scale measure because some are neighbouring. This has implications for reliability investigations because inter-operator disagreements between neighbouring areas are not as serious as disagreements between areas at opposite ends of the pitch.

## Independent and dependent variables

Variables are not only classified by their scale of measurement but also by their role within a study. Variables can also be classified as independent or dependent variables (Vincent, 1999: 8–9; Fallowfield *et al.*, 2005: 52–3). Where a variable, A, is hypothesized to have an influence on some dependent variable, B, A is referred to as the independent variable while B is referred to as the dependent variable. Some studies may have several independent variables and several dependent variables. Some students often make the mistake of thinking that categorical variables must be independent variables. This is not always the case. If we hypothesise that a categorical variable such as venue (home or away) influences performance variables then venue is indeed the independent variable. If, on the other hand, we are investigating the impact of distance travelled (km) on match outcomes (classified as wins, draws and losses), distance travelled is the independent variable even though it is numerical. This has implications for the statistical tests used. If we used an analysis of variances test (ANOVA) to compare distances travelled between matches of different outcomes, we are putting the 'cart before the horse'; we are not going to travel a longer route home just because we lost by more goals than usual. Where we hypothesise that distance travelled or some other numerical variables influence match outcome, a test predicting group membership such as discriminant function analysis would be better.

## TYPES OF DATA PROCESSING

### Elementary statistics

Sports performance data can be analysed using elementary statistics in the same way that data in other areas can. Descriptive statistics can be used within a reductive quantitative approach to determine averages for performance variables, such as the means and medians, as well as describing variability of samples about these averages using standard deviations, ranges or inter-quartile ranges. Relationships between numerical performance variables can be assessed using correlation techniques. Inferential statistical tests are used to express the significance of any differences in the mean (or median) values between samples. Statistical significance is typically represented by a p value which is the probability of a Type I Error. This is the probability that a difference between sub-groups of our sample of performances exists in the wider relevant population of performances from which the sample was drawn. The smaller this probability, the more significant the difference is: $p < 0.05$ means that the probability of making a mistake when claiming the difference according to the sample represents a difference in the wider population is less than 0.05. If $p < 0.001$ then the probability of making such a sampling error is even lower and hence the result is more significant. Although a difference may be highly significant ($p < 0.001$ for example), this simply means that we are 99.9 per cent confident that the difference represents a real difference in the population. This significant difference, that we are confident about, might be a very small difference in real sports terms. Therefore, many researchers also use effect sizes to represent the meaningfulness of the difference. Effect sizes usually represent differences in terms of the variability within the variables used.

These samples compared by inferential statistical tests could compare different independent performances of interest or performances related to the same group of performers. Non-parametric techniques have been

4

used in sports performance analysis research owing to sports performance variables often violating the assumptions of the more powerful parametric procedures.

## Temporal analysis

Many investigations of sports performance provide information in the form of event frequencies and the percentage of events that are performed successfully. Such analysis does not provide important details of temporal orderings of events within sports competitions. Temporal analysis is used to investigate such orderings of events allowing sequences of behaviours to be analysed, providing information on tactics and options used by high level performers in different situations. A simple type of temporal analysis is the use of chi square tests of independence to determine if events are independent of previous events performed within competitions (O'Donoghue and Brown, 2009). The Wald Wolfowitz runs test can be used with dichotomous variables to analyse sequences of events to investigate the concept of momentum in sports performance (Rees and James, 2006). The runs test considers the retrospective probability of success and failure (for example) when performing events and from this determines the expected number of runs of events with the same outcome. If the actual observed number of runs is lower than expected, then the runs are longer runs than would be expected for the given probability of successfully performing an event. This could be evidence of momentum with event outcome being influenced by the outcome of previous events. Another form of temporal analysis is T-pattern analysis. T-pattern analysis involves identifying repeated sequences of events within chronologically ordered event lists. T-patterns (Borrie *et al.*, 2002) have been used in the analysis of soccer (Magnusson, 2000; Bloomfield *et al.*, 2005; Sarmento *et al.*, 2013) and basketball (Lapresa *et al.*, 2013) performance.

## Discriminant function analysis

Discriminant function analysis is a statistical classification technique that attempts to predict group membership using numerical variables. For example, we might wish to model how these numerical variables predict performance outcomes such as wins, draws and losses. Previous matches can be analysed allowing discriminant functions to be produced in terms of the numerical variables. The number of discriminant functions produced is either the number of numerical variables or one less than the number of groups, whichever is less. This means that using three numerical predictor variables to predict whether matches are wins, draws or losses will produce two discriminant functions. Discriminant function analysis also produces a 'territorial map' where the discriminant functions are plotted against each other with areas of the map used to represent different groupings. These groupings could be won matches, drawn matches and lost matches. An alternative to discriminant function analysis that can be used when predicting membership of one of two groups is binary logistic regression. This could be used to examine variables that distinguish between match outcomes where one team (or individual) must win, for example knockout tournament matches in soccer (or tennis).

## Predictive modelling using linear regression

Linear regression can be used in predictive modelling of sports performance. The main difference between linear regression and discriminant function analysis is that discriminant function analysis limits the outcome of matches to broad outcome classes such as win, draw or loss. Linear regression is used to model numerical variables such as the margin of victory in goals or points. Linear regression has been used to model performance in international soccer (O'Donoghue, 2006b) and rugby union (O'Donoghue and Williams, 2004). Performance in these sports is difficult to predict, especially in soccer, even when analysis of previous matches shows some numerical variables, such as ranking points, to be significant predictors. Such variables may be significantly associated with margin of victory on average, but individual match results are not predictable; in international soccer, fewer than 50 per cent of matches are won by the higher ranked of the two teams involved with the remaining results being draws or losses. However, linear-regression based simulation models can be used to study tournaments showing the likelihood of different teams winning. As we will see in Chapter 7, such models show that tournaments such as the FIFA (Fédération Internationale de Football Association) World Cup are wide open with no one team having more than a 25 per cent chance of winning the tournament. Simulation models can also be used in tournament design to

6

show the impact of different tournament structures on the chances of higher ranked teams winning (O'Donoghue, 2005a). Questions about tournaments can be asked and simulation studies used to provide answers. For example, what difference would it make if seeding was not used in a Grand Slam tennis tournament? What would be the difference in soccer ties in domestic cup competitions being completed as single matches or as two legged (home and away) ties. What are the chances of higher ranked teams winning knockout tournaments, round-robin tournaments or hybrid tournaments? Simulation can provide probabilistic information that allows tournament organisers to be better informed when making decisions about tournament structures.

**Cluster analysis**

Sports performers can be grouped according to positional role, gender, level and age group. Similarly, sports performances can be distinguished by conditions such as venue, playing surface, importance of the match and quality of opposition (Taylor *et al.*, 2008; Gomez *et al.*, 2013). However, there are other groupings of performers and performances that are not distinguished by directly observable variables. For example, score-line may influence the tactics used by different players in different ways (O'Donoghue, 2003). Cluster analysis allows non-obvious groupings of players and performances to be identified. Cluster analysis has been used in market research to identify different types of people with respect to product preference (Punj and Stewart, 1983). These groupings can then be analysed with respect to age, gender and socio-economic breakdowns in order to inform marketing strategies. The approach has potential in sports performance analysis as different types of opponent can be recognised and studied allowing more specific preparation for different types of match.

**Principle components analysis**

Principle components analysis has been used in sports performance analysis to reduce large numbers of observed performance variables to a smaller set of broader performance dimensions. If we commence with K performance variables, principle components analysis produces K components that together represent the variability in the data but where some components are worth more than one original variable and others are worth less than a single variable. A majority of the variance in the data can be represented by fewer than one third of the components. These extracted components can then be used in a more concise analysis of the data than if the original variables were used. However, there are two concerns with the use of principle components with sports performance analysis. First, the originally recorded performance variables may be clearly understood by practitioners whereas the principle components are Z scores with no units and no norms for interpretation. Second, the principle components are not universal performance variables but are variables produced from the data that the principle components analysis was applied to. There may be correlations (or lack of correlation) between pairs of variables in the dataset that is analysed that would not be found more generally. Despite these concerns, principle components analysis can be used to identify correlated performance variables that represent the same broad dimensions of performance. This information could then be used to identify critical subsets of data to be used in live analysis systems where it is not possible to gather full performance data.

## Artificial Intelligence

Computers are much better than humans at dealing with large volumes of data and performing well defined tasks at high speeds. For example, a human would not be expected to accurately remember and recall the telephone numbers of everyone in the country. Humans, on the other hand, are better than computers when understanding and utilising more complex data. For example, voice recognition and face recognition tasks can be performed almost instantaneously by humans but are still major research areas for the computer science community. The broad area of computer science where complex data and tasks requiring human-like intelligence are required is called Artificial Intelligence.

Many types of data in sports performance are complex patterns of information rather than well-defined numerical performance indicators. In many areas, including geology (Bugaets et al., 1991) and medicine (Szolovits, 1982), artificial intelligence has been used to analyse complex data. Lapham and Bartlett (1995) reviewed artificial intelligence techniques with potential use in biomechanics and sports performance analysis. Despite the potential application areas in sports performance

8

analysis, Bartlett (2004) conceded that since Latham and Bartlett's (1995) review had been published developments were limited. Technique analysis had used artificial neural networks; specifically, Kohonen self-organising maps had been used in the analysis of javelin throw, discuss throw and soccer kicking technique while multi-layered neural networks had been used in the analysis of shot-put technique (Bartlett, 2004). More recent research into artificial neural networks has been published about their application in technique analysis (Lamb and Bartlett, 2013) and tactical movement patterns in game sports (Perl *et al.*, 2013). However, other areas of artificial intelligence, such as expert systems and genetic algorithms, have still to be exploited in sports performance analysis (Bartlett, 2004).

## Data mining

Data mining has been described by Frawley *et al.* (1991) as 'the non-trivial extraction of important, previously unknown and potentially useful information from data'. This goes beyond simple database querying and statistical analysis. Data mining integrates the areas of database technology, statistics, high performance algorithms, machine learning, mathematics and visualisation. Data mining has been used to identify valuable marketing information in sectors such as retail (Shaw *et al.*, 2001). However, there are some criticisms of data mining for knowledge discovery in sports performance. First, the use of high performance algorithms is not a priority where the value of the information produced justifies an overnight run of data mining algorithms. Data mining exercises are typically one-off studies rather than routine database queries that are frequently used. While the automatic searching for potential patterns of interest within the data has yielded valuable knowledge in various domains, it can be criticised for lacking direction. Analyses that are not directed by clear hypotheses have been criticized: 'the baroness of multivariate data grubbing' (Kirk-Smith, 1998). Therefore, analysis of large sports performance datasets have typically been framed by specifying hypotheses and then utilising the necessary data mining tools and techniques in order to answer questions posed of the data. This is not a pure automatic data mining approach but does involve the stages of data cleaning, extraction, analysis and presentation performed in data mining. There are additional stages that are included when mining sports performance data. For example, performance aggregation is where data from individual performances of players are used to produce an overall performance record for the player to be utilised during analysis (O'Donoghue, 2006a).

## STAGES OF DATA PROCESSING

Figure 1.1 shows the six broad stages of handling data described by Graham (1991). The first stage of posing the question is important as it dictates the purpose of the analysis and what is required. This should be considered carefully in order to determine the data to be collected and analysed as well as the output information needed. Any data processing activity should be well designed before data gathering commences in academic and practical contexts. Projects that are unsuccessful often fail because those undertaking them do not have a clear purpose, do not know why they are collecting the data they are gathering and do not know where the study is going. The purpose of the study dictates the goal post of the analysis. Graham (1991) refers to this as the question. The question is not just a purpose of the study, but a framework into which the answer will fit. The question guides the analysis of data because we

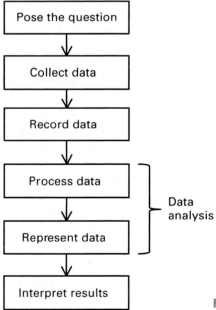

Figure 1.1 Stages of data processing

know that the resulting information is specifically intended to answer the question. The collecting and recording of data appear to be the same task, but there is a subtle difference. An observer could observe sports performance and come to conclusions based on what they have memorised in the short or longer term. Even where data are being recorded, some observed data might not be stored. For example, a manual system that uses tallying to record the frequency of different event types will lose information about temporal orderings of events. It is also possible to create computerised systems that accumulate frequencies without recording the raw data as they are entered. This is very rare in systems developed nowadays because of advances in disk storage technology and a dramatic reduction in cost. Data are processed and summarised effectively as output information that can then be interpreted to support decisions being made by the consumers of system outputs. Graham (1991) referred to the combined stages of data processing and representation as data analysis.

## DAVIDSON'S (1996) PRINCIPLES OF DATA HANDLING

While writing this book the authors reviewed available textbooks dealing with data analysis in sport and more generally. It had already been decided to make the first chapter about principles of data processing when the book proposal was submitted to the publisher. During the review of available textbooks on data processing, Davidson's (1996) book on data handling became particularly relevant. Davidson's book discussed 30 principles of data processing in educational contexts. Most of the principles are highly relevant to sports performance analysis and are examples of the advice that the authors have typically given to students undertaking practical and academic work in recent years. This section of the current chapter describes 25 of Davidson's 30 principles that are most relevant to sports performance analysis.

### The atomicity principle (Davidson, 1996: 9–10)

The atomicity principle is that you cannot analyse below the level at which the data were observed. For example, if we have gathered data on possessions in a team game without classifying them as being restarts or possession changes during open play, then we will not be able to analyse these different types of possessions. Those developing sports perform-ance analysis systems should consider the ways in which the data could be analysed. If we gather data on different types of possession but find that some types are very rare, we can combine these possession classes during later analysis. This is analysing above the level at which the data were observed. The case for distinguishing between different possession types as much as possible during data collection is that a possession type needs to be entered for each event anyway. Classifying possessions by type, therefore, does not add to the volume of data collection and does give the option to combine possession types during analysis if necessary.

### The appropriate data principle (Davidson, 1996: 10–11) and the data control principle (Davidson, 1996: 32)

The appropriate data principle and the data control principle are related. The appropriate data principle is that you cannot analyse what you have not measured. This may seem obvious, but it does have implications for the requirements analysis phase of system development. The data control principle is that analysts should take control of the structure of data and how data are processed. System developers should gain the fullest possi-ble understanding of the information to be provided when analysing data and the types of data processing query to be served. An issue related to data control is version control. This may arise from redundant copies of data, especially where multiple analysts are involved. One analyst might update one version of the data while another analyst updates another copy of the data. When either data set is analysed, we will have outputs or intermediate results for an incorrect or incomplete data set. This can result in having to take data right back to the original data set and redo the updates, amendments and analyses in sequence. The best way to avoid such problems is to have version control policies.

### The social consequences principle (Davidson, 1996: 12–15)

The social consequences principle is that data about individuals are used in decision-making processes that can affect those individuals. In sports performance analysis, data are used to evaluate player performances, when selecting squads and in scouting. The main clients requiring deci-sion making information are coaches and high performance directors

# 12

(Wiltshire, 2013) as well as players who can learn from feedback provided. The data need to be valid and reliable to ensure that important decisions are well informed (O'Donoghue and Longville, 2004). Data need to be thoroughly checked before being used in analysis. This can delay the time at which the data become available, but where accuracy is important this is justified. For example, during live data entry for a soccer match, the entry of a player performing a tackle might be less than 100 per cent accurate. Individual player tackling statistics could be discussed with players during debriefings. Therefore, processes need to be put in place to allow video sequences of tackles performed by each player to be checked with event data altered if necessary. Today's interactive video feedback systems allow for efficient checking.

**Two laws of computing: back it up, do it now! (Davidson, 1996: 15)**

Data processing can be very efficient, especially when done by computerised systems. Data gathering, on the other hand, can be highly laborious. Raw data need to be backed up immediately and many commercial video analysis systems continually save video files and event databases as they are being operated so that the data will survive on disk in the event of a power failure. Data files can be backed up on cloud storage, on multiple hard drives and emailed to the analyst's own email address as an attachment for additional backup.

**The data efficiency principle (Davidson, 1996: 42)**

The data efficiency principle is that data should be collected efficiently but not at the cost of losing crucial data. There can be compromises between efficient data gathering and efficient data analysis when using manual notation systems. However, computerised packages allow efficient data analysis meaning that developers of systems and processes should concentrate on making data entry as efficient as possible. This has implications for the ergonomic aspects of hardware used, the interface of software packages and for the structure of data entry tasks that need to reflect operators' mental models of sports performance being observed. Data entry should consider data processing tasks to ensure that data are collected in a form that is readily usable by analysis packages. For example, where data is to be loaded into SPSS from Microsoft Excel for statistical analysis, there must be one row per case, one column for each variable or repeated measure of a variable and a single row of headings. Where data are entered without considering required formats for analysis packages to be used, time is wasted transforming the data into the correct structure. The most infuriating thing about this is that entering the data in the correct format in the first place may have been easier to do than entering the data in an incorrect format.

### The data manipulation principle (Davidson, 1996: 57)

The data manipulation principle is to let computers do as much of the processing work as possible. In sports performance analysis, this can start as data are being gathered. There are activation links in packages such as Sportscode where user-entered events automatically trigger higher order events. Sportscode also has a Statistical Window that can be programmed to produce information from the events entered. This saves users a great deal of time. When data are exported from any sports performance analysis package, they can be analysed efficiently to produce other variables. For example, score-line states can be determined from the data entered and events satisfying given criteria can be identified.

### The original data principle (Davidson, 1996: 61)

The original data principle is to always save a copy of the original unaltered data. If we start processing data, altering it as we do so, when we make mistakes we may not be able to reproduce the original data to analyse it. It is easy enough to save an additional copy of the data file before processing commences. This can mean that we have redundant copies of the data where the data are included as the starting point in spreadsheet files where processing is done. However, computer disk storage is relatively inexpensive, allowing redundant copies to be made quickly and without having to delete other files. Storing a copy of the original data not only means storing the content of all data records but also preserving the order of records. The chronological order of event records may be important to some types of analyses to be done.

14

## The Kludge principle (Davidson, 1996: 64)

The Kludge principle states that the most elegant way to manipulate data is not always the best way. The author of the current chapter did an undergraduate degree in computer science in the early 1980s where students were taught how to improve the efficiency of algorithms taking into consideration storage requirements and CPU usage. There are processor-intensive applications as well as storage-intensive application areas where these issues should still be addressed. However, for most sports performance data analysis, processing can be done in steps saving the intermediate data produced at each step. For example, we could commence with the raw data on one worksheet in Microsoft Excel, copying it into another worksheet for the first stage of analysis. The data and new data within this and successive worksheets can be copied into new worksheets to perform subsequent stages of the analysis. Preserving the intermediate data produced at different stages allows checking before proceeding to the next stage of the analysis. A further point is that some 'elegant' data processing techniques might not be naturally understandable to all analysts. The Kludge principle allows analysts to process the data in smaller more understandable steps.

## The default principle (Davidson, 1996: 66)

The default principle is that those collecting and analysing data should be aware of the default settings of any software used. For example, when entering value labels in Sportscode, we can choose for these to appear in all currently active events being recorded or only in the most recent event started by the user. The way in which data are recorded depends on the settings of the system being used during recording. If operators are not aware of the current settings of software, there is a danger that they could gather data for an entire performance before realising that the data have not been recorded as intended.

## The complex data structure principle (Davidson, 1996: 78)

The complex data structure principle states that if we can use complex data structures then we should use them. Much sports performance data are stored in the form of two-dimensional tables where we have event records containing different fields for event variables such as the team performing the event, time of the event, event type, location and outcome. There are occasions where multi-dimensional arrays of event records would be preferable. For example, if dealing with player tracking data, we might want to address a player's location at some point during the match using the match period (half), time within the match period, team and player within the team. This is a four dimensional array of X–Y player location records. We might also have a store of multiple match player tracking data where further dimensions would help algorithms address particular data in a clearer way than if multiple conceptual dimensions were mapped onto a single artificial dimension (using Iliffe Vectors for example). The case of player tracking data is interesting when we consider that substitutions can be made and players can be dismissed. We also have squads of players with different subsets of players competing in different matches. Data structures, therefore, need to represent who played in each match and at what times they were playing within the matches.

Variant records allow different event types to have different fields of data. For example, records for net points in tennis might need data about the cause of approaching the net (drawn in, drop shot, approach shot, etc.) and the outcome of approaching the net (volley winner, volley error, passed, lobbed, etc.) that do not need to be recorded for other point types.

**The impossibility/implausibility principle (Davidson, 1996: 118)**

The impossibility/implausibility principle is that we should identify any event records that have recorded data that must be erroneous. This can be done very efficiently by programming conditional functions to access fields from records determining the truth of whether the data satisfy data integrity constraints. One of the first stages of 'data mining' is data cleaning where such errors are identified and corrected before processing the data further. For example, we may record the number of shots played in a tennis rally including the serve, who won the point and whether the point was won with a winner or an opponent error. There are 8 ($2 \times 2 \times 2$) combinations of point winner (serving or receiving player), shots played (odd or even number) and point outcome (winner or error), four of which are impossible. One of these errors is that the server has won the point with a winner and there was an even number of shots played.

16

It could be that the receiver actually won the point, or that there were an odd number of shots played or that the outcome was an opponent error. Detecting that an error has occurred does not diagnose the exact error. However, it does allow us to go back to match video and check or delete the entire point record. The Boolean conditional functions used to detect such errors can be pasted into thousands of rows very quickly with rows then being sorted so that all of the erroneous point records are located together in the data set for the purpose of data cleaning. There are other simpler checks such as all percentage variables should be between 0 and 100. Other errors might not be within single event records but between pairs or sequences of records within a data set. For example, if we have a team scoring a goal in a soccer match, the most recent previous event where a team took possession of the ball must have been for the scoring team. If this between-records constraint is violated then an error has been made that can be detected by programming conditions for recognising such an error.

### The extant error principle (Davidson, 1996: 122) and the manual check principle (Davidson, 1996: 122)

The extant error principle assumes that errors exist and should be actively looked for. Results should be checked for unexpected outcomes and the data analysis process checked to see whether these outputs are correct, which they might be, or not. For example, when the authors first developed a Matlab simulator to predict the 2014 FIFA World Cup (Chapter 7), there were several teams winning more of the 20,000 simulated World Cup tournaments than Spain despite Spain being the highest ranked team. The progression statistics were as expected for the group stages of the tournament but not for the knockout stages. This observation was the starting point of the debugging process that led to an error being identified and corrected. Analysts can use synthetic data to test for different types of error they suspect of being present. A manual check is what software engineers refer to as a dry run. This is where they write down some input values and then consider data processing functions, applying them to the values to determine the intermediate data produced at various stages of the process and to determine the final outputs that would be produced by the process for the given input data.

### The error typology principle (Davidson, 1996: 129)

The error typology principle states that analysts should classify errors as they discover them. For example: there are 3 broad classes of data entry error in match analysis (James *et al.*, 2002); definitional errors, perceptual errors and data entry errors. Definitional errors are where event types are vaguely defined, meaning operators do not share the same understanding of their meaning. Perceptual errors are where operators understand event definitions but misclassify particular events. For example, an event might be performed on the border of two areas of the playing surface and the operator has to enter one or the other. Data entry errors are where an operator has correctly recognised an event but pressed the wrong key during data entry. There are additional processing errors that occur after data entry. Syntax and semantic errors are flagged during the development of processing tools and so are easily identified. Logical errors are more serious because computerised systems will simply execute the instructions set by analysts. A logical error is where a processing function is coded incorrectly or accesses incorrect data. Expressions with several pairs of parentheses and functions with nested IF statements are easy to enter incorrectly and analysts are encouraged to use smaller processing steps to make the instructions and functions clearer.

### The know yourself principle (Davidson, 1996: 149)

The know yourself principle is that analysts should understand the types of questions they ask of data. In sports performance analysis, analysts need to have an understanding of the types of analysis required by the coaches and athletes they work with. An understanding of these analyses allows processes to be rehearsed so that analysts can give timescales to coaches for when required information can be available after data are collected.

### The correlative data principle (Davidson, 1996: 155)

The correlative data principle warns against doing straightforward analyses on data just because they can be done easily. We may have 20 variables meaning that $(20 \times (20-1) / 2 = )$ 190 pairs of variables can be correlated. However, some of these correlations may be meaningless and are not worth inspecting. Instead, it would be better to focus analysis around hypothesised independent and dependent variables or hypothesised relationships between variables. For example, in a study of tennis performance, we may have a clear research question comparing performance between women's and men's singles matches. Comparing values for 19 remaining variables between women's and men's singles matches gives a more focused and concise analysis of 19 results rather than 190 speculative comparisons.

**The expected data principle (Davidson, 1996: 157)**

The expected data principle states that we should modify data, while retaining a copy of the original data, in order to specifically produce the required results. For example, we may have ten different types of set piece in a sport, but could merge them into three broader types of set piece for the purpose of providing required output. We have 16 different point scores within tennis games if we consider all Deuce points to be the same, 30–40 to be the same as Advantage Receiver and 40–30 to be the same as Advantage Server. With so many point types, some may occur too infrequently to allow stable data to be gathered. Therefore, points could be classified into three broad types: game points for the server, break points for the receiver, or other points. Very often in data analysis exercises we devise processes by considering the purpose of the analysis, the results format that conveys what will be found most clearly and the format of the data that have been collected. This gives direction to the analysis process.

**The unit of observation principle**

The unit of observation principle states that the unit of observation is not always the most appropriate unit of analysis. For example, we may record data about individual passes in a game of soccer. There is actually a choice of unit of analysis that can be applied to the data. We could use the pass event as the unit of analysis comparing successful passes made by our team with unsuccessful passes. There may be other factors such as period of the match or area of the pitch that are associated with the proportion of successful passes made. This allows a computerised video analysis system to be used to interactively review video sequences of unsuccessful passes. In an academic study, we may have data from many soccer matches meaning that matches, team performances, player performances, teams or players could be used as the units of analysis. Chapter 8 on non-parametric statistical tests explains how statistical significance can be achieved by analysing at an individual event level. However, while there may be hundreds or thousands of passes in the data set, these may have come from fewer than six matches that may not be representative of soccer performance in general. Player performances within matches can include a numerical variable which is the percentage of passes that are successful. This can also be done for team performances within matches. Teams and players can also be considered over the course of a season representing their percentage of passes that are successful over the season. The percentage variables are derived from the individual pass event data that are recorded.

**The reinventing the wheel principle (Davidson, 1996: 206)**

The reinventing the wheel principle would be better named the 'avoid reinventing the wheel principle' because Davidson was advocating archiving successful procedures. Microsoft Excel allows macros to be recorded so that they can be reused on further data. Reinventing the wheel can also be avoided by knowing what software packages are capable of. Things like absolute addressing of cells with the '$' character in Excel, pivot tables, table lookup functions and macros can be extremely useful. Very often analysts reinvent the wheel because they do not take the time to investigate useful features of packages like Microsoft Excel. The short-term investment in skill development can lead to much greater time savings in the long term.

**The save output principle (Davidson, 1996: 213) and the regenerative output principle (Davidson, 1996: 214)**

The save output principle and the regenerative output principle are connected and in many situations we apply one principle or the other depending on how long it takes to reproduce output. If analyses can be applied to stored data very quickly then there is not as much need to store the output as there is when performing the analysis is more time consuming. There are also educational reasons for not storing outputs of analyses done in practical sessions of research process and data analysis modules. It would be far better for students to be able to repeat data analyses rather than have a collection of output files stored without understanding how they were produced or why.

### The know your system principle (Davidson, 1996: 214)

The know your system principle is about analysts understanding the constraints and limitations of the systems with which they are working. This includes speed of processing, storage capacity, battery capacities and quirks of the system. Analysts often need to know the resolution of video that can be captured live under different operating conditions. For example, if the system is transferring video footage live through a wired link to an output screen on the coach's bench, this will require extra CPU usage that might result in frames being lost. The knowledge of system constraints and limitations allows analysts to advise coaches about the trade-offs between video resolution and frequency of dropped frames during video capture under different operating conditions.

### The output = data principle (Davidson, 1996: 217) and the output = input principle (Davidson, 1996: 217)

The output = data and output = input principles are related to each other. Data processing activities can be structured into pipelines of processes where the output from one process is the input to some other process. Data are input into an analysis process that produces summary information as output. For example, in Excel we can use a pivot table to cross-tabulate players with event types. The cross-tabulated frequencies can then be used to determine the percentage of events performed by each player that were of each type.

### SUMMARY

Data analysis in sports performance analysis has much in common with data analysis in other fields. Davidson's (1996) principles of data handling are applicable in sports performance analysis and experienced analysts will be familiar with the principles even if they have never read Davidson's book. Data analyses applied to sports performance data include statistical analysis, temporal analysis, artificial neural networks, modelling, simulation and data mining.

# CHAPTER 2

## ANALYSIS FACILITIES OF COMMERCIAL PACKAGES

### INTRODUCTION

This chapter covers the basic analysis features provided by commercial sports performance analysis systems. There are packages that typically are used for match analysis dealing with broad events within game sports. These packages include Focus X2, Nacsport, Sportscode, Dartfish and Observer Pro. The main analysis process of such packages involves cross-tabulating variables to provide frequency profiles. There are other packages, such as Silicon Coach, used in the analysis of technique during shorter-term events. The main analysis facilities of these systems are distance and angle estimation functions. Some systems such as Dartfish and Focus X3 can be used for both match analysis and analysis of technique. Analysis of technique will be covered in a separate textbook within this series. Therefore, this chapter concentrates on the analysis features of match analysis systems. Three particular packages are used as exemplars when describing the types of data analysis facilities available.

### FOCUS X2

Focus X2 (Elite Sports Analysis, Delgaty Bay, Fife, Scotland) abstracts events as being performed instantaneously with a duration of zero seconds. For example, a pass in football could be represented as the point in time when a player's foot struck the ball. The user defines a pre-roll period and a post-roll period to be used if the event is to be shown as a video clip. The pre-roll is the period before the event and the post-roll is the period after the event. The amount of pre-roll and post-roll to be set for an event type depends on the amount of video that the user wishes to see when replaying the event. The pre-roll and post-roll need to be long enough to allow the cause and consequences of events to be viewed and short enough so that briefing sessions using the video sequences can be efficient. Focus X2 also allows the video to play on from the time of the event rather than defining a specific post-roll. This is useful for event types where the amount of video users need to see varies between occurrences of the event type. For example, in a team game we could have an event 'possession', which starts as soon as a team takes possession of the ball. The possession ends when the team scores or loses the ball. Some possessions last longer than others and so we would not wish to impose a uniform post-roll on all possessions.

Events are represented by a record consisting of values for relevant variables. For example, possessions in soccer might be represented by the following variables:

■ Team – the team who are in possession of the ball.
■ Period – the section of the match in which the possession occurred.
■ Type – the method by which the team came to be in possession of the ball.
■ Start location – the part of the playing area where the possession started.
■ Number of passes.
■ End location – the part of the playing area where the possession ended.
■ Outcome – how the possession ended.

Commercial video analysis packages are generic and can be tailored for use with sports or activities of the user's choice. This is achieved by using metadata to define the sport. Metadata are data about data. Focus X2 uses a Category Set to define a sport in terms of the events of interest and the data to be recorded about these events. A Category Set is composed of categories that represent the variables of interest (for example: team, period, type of possession, start location, number of passes, end location and outcome). When an event is entered, a value is needed for each of the categories. The Category Set contains buttons representing the values of each category. For example, the category Team could have two values,

'Home team' and 'Away team'. Figure 2.1 shows the Category Set for the possession example.

When the system is in 'logging mode', the Category Set is used to enter events into the Event List. We create an event by choosing one value from each category. The event is timed on one category and logged on another. This preserves the time of the possession while the user enters values for the other categories. For example, in the possession analysis system, possessions are timed on the Team event and logged on the Outcome event. This is denoted by the stopwatch and diamond symbols respectively. Readers with experience of computerised match analysis will realise that this is a challenging system to operate live. As one possession ends with an interception, the user needs to enter data about the number of passes that have been counted, the location where the possession ended and the fact that it ended with the ball being intercepted by

| Category | Values | | | | | | | | | | |
|---|---|---|---|---|---|---|---|---|---|---|---|
| Team (○) | Home team | | | | | Away team | | | | | |
| Period | Quarter 1 | | | Quarter 2 | | | Quarter 3 | | | Quarter 4 | | |
| Type | Kick off | | Throw in | | Corner | | Free kick | | Interception | | Tackle | |
| Start Location | Def L | | | | Mid L | | | | Att L | | | |
| | Def C | | | | Mid C | | | | Att C | | | |
| | Def R | | | | Mid R | | | | Att R | | | |
| Number of passes | 0 | 1 | 2 | 3 | 4 | 5 | 6 | 7 | 8 | 9 | 10 | 11+ |
| End Location | Def L | | | | Mid L | | | | Att L | | | |
| | Def C | | | | Mid C | | | | Att C | | | |
| | Def R | | | | Mid R | | | | Att R | | | |
| Outcome (♦) | Goal | | Shot on target | | Shot off target | | Ball out of play | | Tackled | Interception | | Free conceded |

Figure 2.1 A category set in Focus X2

Notes: (○ The stopwatch symbol is used to represent the category on which the event is timed, ♦ the diamond symbol is used to represent the category that logs the event)

the opponents. While the user has been pressing these buttons, the next possession will have already started. Therefore, the system can only be operated live by a highly skilled user and with a sufficient pre-roll because the user will have reacted to the start of a possession some seconds after the possession actually commenced. We will assume that the system is not operated live and that video pausing is used to ensure each possession is tagged at the point at which it starts. In between selecting a value for the variable that the event is timed on and a value for the variable that the event is logged on, the user can change the values entered for any of the other variables until they are correct. The system only completes and stores the event record when a value is entered for the variable that the event is logged on. In the possession analysis example, the user positions the variable at the start of the possession and enters a value for Team to time the event. Values for the other variables except Outcome are then entered to create the event record. One exception to this is where 'sticky buttons' are used. A sticky button is useful where a category's value is usually the same as it was for the previous event. For example, the Period in which possessions occur is Quarter 1 until the analysis gets to the second quarter. Setting Period up so that the value buttons are sticky buttons means that the previously used Period value (the given quarter) will remain selected as a default when the next possession commences. This saves the user having to enter the same value for Period in successive possessions.

Once all of the possessions in the match have been entered during 'logging mode' in Focus X2, the system can be switched to 'review mode' so that the events can be analysed. The interface of the Focus X2 package consists of a video player, the Category Set, the Event List and a Results Grid. Not all events in the Event List can be shown at once, so a scroll bar is used. Figure 2.1 illustrates how the Category Set is used in review mode. The Category Set is used to set criteria for the events we wish to focus in on for video replay or quantitative analysis. This is done by selecting any values of any categories that apply. In this example, the user wishes to see those possessions of the Home Team that contained six or more passes that resulted in a scoring opportunity (goal, shot on target or shot off target) in Quarter 3 and Quarter 4. The user is not concerned about start location, end location or the type of possession and so all of the values of these three categories apply. Once the user has established criteria such as these, the Event List will only include those events that satisfy those criteria.

26

The Results Grid can be used to cross-tabulate pairs of categories. For example, we could cross-tabulate Type of possession and Team to compare the frequency profile of possession types between the two teams. Users can choose to apply the Results Grid to all recorded events or just to the events satisfying the criteria expressed in the Category Set. The latter option is useful for obtaining specific results. For example, if we wished to see the outcomes of different possessions for a single team, we would select that team, deselect the other team and make sure all values were selected for the remaining categories. Then the Results Grid could cross-tabulate Type of possession and Outcome just for that team. This can be done for each team in turn. Other restrictions, such as match periods of interest, can also be used to limit the events (possessions in this case) that are considered when viewing the Results Grid.

The Results Grid is limited to providing frequencies of events. Where we are interested in timings of different event types, we can export the entire Event List into Microsoft Excel and then use a pivot table to determine the mean duration of possessions of different outcomes performed by the two teams. This use of Excel will be described in detail in Chapter 3. Focus X2 supports qualitative analysis of video sequences by coaches and players. The Category Set can be used to establish criteria for video sequences of interest and then these can be played at normal speed or slow motion, with pausing and replaying being used.

## SPORTSCODE

Sportscode uses a Code Window to show the events that can be recorded using the system. Main events are recorded using code buttons and extra metadata can be provided in the form of text labels. Sportscode (Sportstec Inc., Warriewood, New South Wales, Australia) differs from Focus X2 in two main ways. First, events in Sportscode can have a non-zero duration with differing start time and end times. Events of a given event type can have varying durations depending on when the operator chooses to record the end of events. Events may be exclusively linked with other events meaning that the start of one event can deactivate an existing event that is being recorded. The second difference to Focus X2 is that Sportscode uses a timeline, which is a graphical representation of behaviours that have been tagged. The timeline can be exported as an Event List for further processing if needed. The events in Sportscode typically have duration with lead times and lag times being used to store the duration of the event (start time to end time) within the timeline. It is technically possible to have some instantaneous events in Sportscode where lead time and lag time are set to 0s. This would, however, only display a single frame for the event but could be useful for marking events that are not to be shown as video clips.

Sportscode uses value label buttons to record other information about events. An advantage over Focus X2 is that we are not forced to use categories with a value being entered for each category. Some event types might require more labels than others. This can only be accomplished in Focus X2 by using a 'N/A' (not applicable) value within categories that are used with a subset of event types. Instances of events in the timeline can be manipulated directly by the user (with the mouse) allowing the video sequence to be shown or the instance can be dragged into a movie organiser window used to create a highlights movie.

There are three ways of using the Code Window; edit mode, coding mode and labelling mode. Edit mode is used to create the Code Window in the first place and coding mode is used for data entry during the match, or during post-match analysis or a combination of both. Labelling mode is used when the events have been entered into the timeline but there is some additional labelling of events to be done that could not have been done when the video was originally tagged. Once the events are entered into the timeline and any additional labelling of events has been done, the data can be analysed. The main analysis facilities provided by Sportscode are:

- the Matrix;
- row operations;
- the sorter window;
- the Statistical Window.

Programming a Statistical Window to analyse the data in the timeline is the subject of Chapter 5 and so will not be discussed any further in the current chapter.

The Matrix facility of Sportscode will be illustrated using the same example of possession analysis that was used to illustrate Focus X2. In this implementation of the system, there are two sets of buttons representing the six event types. The first set of buttons is for the six events when

# 28

being performed by the home team and the second set of buttons is for the six events when being performed by the away team. These buttons have activation links to buttons for the specific events and activation links to labels for the home and away team. The advantage of this is that when an event occurs, the user only needs to press one button rather than two for both the team and event type to be recorded. There are also activation links from the value label buttons for individual outcome types to two broader classes of outcome ('Opportunity' and 'No opportunity'). All possession type events associated with teams (12 of them) are mutually exclusive as are the six possession type events that they activate. Figure 2.2 shows the layout of the Code Window. There are 37 different value labels. These can be formed into a label tree to make post-match

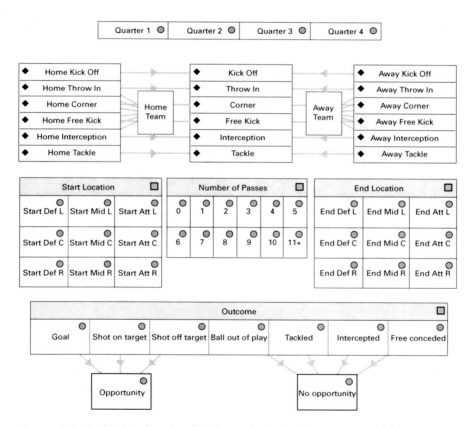

Figure 2.2 Code Window for the SportsCode implementation of the possession analysis system

labelling of events easier. Instead of being presented with a single list of 37 labels, we can initially be presented with options for match period, start location, number of passes, end location and outcome. We can choose one of these and then be presented with a sub-menu of value labels for the given label group.

The Matrix is the main analysis feature of Sportscode and shows a cross-tabulation of events and labels. The Matrix Organiser facility of earlier versions of Sportscode allowed users to select value labels or combinations of value labels to include in the event by label matrix displayed. In more recent versions of Sportscode, the Matrix Organiser facility has been merged with the standard matrix facility.

The Matrix can be accessed from the timeline or the Code Window. Once it is opened, some unwanted columns can be deleted from the Matrix. The '+' button on the top right hand side of the Matrix window can be used to add new columns to represent combinations of value labels. For example, we may want to have a column of the Matrix representing instances when a possession of the away team leads to an opportunity. We click on the '+' button on the top right of the Matrix window and when we are asked to select a value, we can choose 'Away Team'. A new column appears showing the frequency of each possession event performed by the away team. We highlight this column; the function bar at the top of the window shows that the highlighted column includes Away Team. We can now use the '+' button again to add 'Opportunity' to the current column. These will be AND-ed together as a default, meaning the column now lists the frequency of each event type performed by the Away Team where there was a scoring opportunity. We can change the AND to OR or NOT. We are not limited to a single operator. For example, we could have a column that represented any possessions with six or more passes (6 OR 7 OR 8 OR 9 OR 10 OR 11+). Figure 2.3 shows a Matrix where we can see possessions for each team as well as possessions for each team that led to scoring opportunities or not.

Once we have added any new columns representing any combination of value labels that we are interested in to the Matrix, we can save the Matrix as a matrix file, which can be used with further matches without having to redo the process of selecting label combinations again.

In our timeline, we can create new rows which merge existing rows. In the menu bar select **Rows → Create New Row** which causes the Add Row popup window to appear asking us for the name of the new row, which

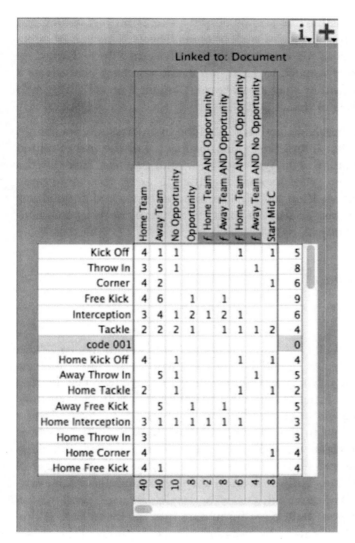

Figure 2.3 A Matrix in SportsCode

rows we wish to combine and whether we wish to combine them with an AND or an OR. For example we could choose Throw Ins and Corners to see statistics for these set pieces combined in the Matrix. We can also use the NOT operator to create a single row that contains instances for all times when some chosen event does not occur.

The data in the timeline can also be output as an Event List, which can be processed in other packages such as spreadsheets. This can be effectively analysed using pivot tables. We can also use **File → Export → Instance Frequency Report**, to set up an event summary analysis as a starting point for further analysis in Excel. Chapter 9 on reliability will provide an example of this.

In considering the analysis facilities provided by Sportscode, we should include the fact that interactive video feedback and the use of edited movies allows qualitative analysis by players and coaches. There are the usual pause, rewind, step forward facilities to assist this more open analysis of the information in the video frames. Notes and annotations can be added and there is also the ability to dictate a coaching commentary onto selected clips.

## DARTFISH TEAM PRO

### Tagging Panel

Dartfish Team Pro (6.0) (Dartfish, Fribourg, Switzerland) has two main functions available for analysis, one allowing technique analysis (Analyser) and the other observational analysis (Tagging). The Tagging function allows the input of data via a Tagging Panel for a team or individual player analysis to be undertaken. Figure 2.4 is an example of a Tagging Panel. When in the Tagging mode of the software, the screen offers sections for video viewing, coding via the Tagging Panel and viewing of the data entered via the Events list. The software has a number of sample Tagging Panels built-in to allow the user to understand the various functionalities of each tool. These Tagging Panels use a combination of Event and Keyword buttons to input data into the Event List, allowing multiple levels of data to be assigned to specific times of the video. The Tagging Panel editor also has a number of layout organisational tools that allow buttons to be grouped together and organised into tab boxes that can be stacked, for an ergonomic design.

Performance variables can be recorded using the Event creation tools of either 'Event' or 'Continuous Event' buttons. Event buttons create an event of fixed duration; this is controlled by the administering of a pre-roll and overall duration. The manner in which this timing works is different to other software, as the overall duration takes into account any

32

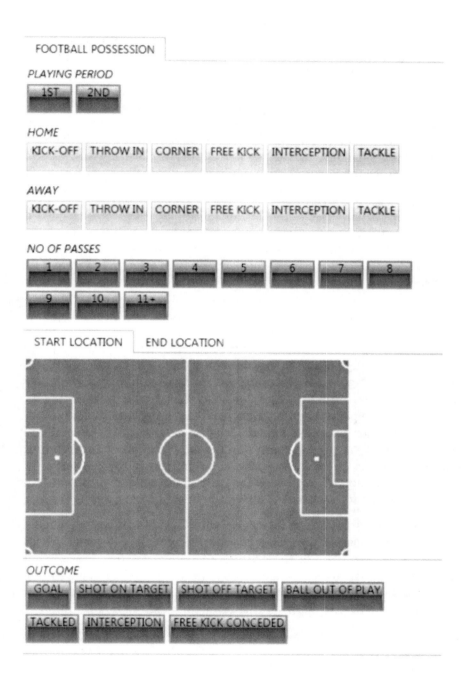

**FOOTBALL POSSESSION**

PLAYING PERIOD

| 1ST | 2ND |

HOME

| KICK-OFF | THROW IN | CORNER | FREE KICK | INTERCEPTION | TACKLE |

AWAY

| KICK-OFF | THROW IN | CORNER | FREE KICK | INTERCEPTION | TACKLE |

NO OF PASSES

| 1 | 2 | 3 | 4 | 5 | 6 | 7 | 8 |

| 9 | 10 | 11+ |

START LOCATION    END LOCATION

OUTCOME

| GOAL | SHOT ON TARGET | SHOT OFF TARGET | BALL OUT OF PLAY |

| TACKLED | INTERCEPTION | FREE KICK CONCEDED |

Figure 2.4 Dartfish Tagging Panel

pre-roll time allocated, i.e. If a button were allocated a duration of ten seconds with a pre-roll of five seconds, the event will include five seconds prior to the moment that it was pressed and five seconds after. It is important to remember this, as this timing controls the section of video each event refers to. Continuous Events allows the event to have an unrestricted duration, in which the user must switch the button on and off. These timings can also be further controlled by administering offset durations to the start and end of the event, allowing for reaction time. These events provide the time-based information and allow for additional data to be attributed to each event via keywords.

Keyword Addition Tools of Keyword Buttons, Persistent Keyword Buttons, Text Box, Score Panel and Zone Tool can record the additional data that provides the extra depth of analysis to these events. Keyword Buttons allow for description of the events. When tagging, keyword data is attributed to the current button. Keywords can also be added post initial analysis via the Events List. A persistent keyword adds this data for the entire duration that it is active. The Text Box tool is a special persistent keyword that allows for basic short text to be added to an event. This is useful when the user wants to add competition data, game location or playing condition details. The score panel has the ability to keep track of score for two teams on a +1/−1 basis and allows for events to categorised based on the current scoring. This tool is not suitable for complex scoring patterns such as that used in tennis. Last, the Zone Tool is a handy tool for recording the pitch location of events. Any pitch image can be added to the Tagging Panel and the number of rows and columns that make up the individual zones can be defined in the properties of this tool. Users don't visually see the demarcation of these zones when tagging, apart from the change of keyword when hovering over the image.

For this keyword data to be included in the Events List and associated with the events tagged, they must be grouped by using categories. These categories are important features for not only the data entry process, but also the data analysis as Category titles are then used to compare the tagging data via tables. Without these grouping categories, the only columns in the Events List would be Number, Position and Duration.

An added feature of Dartfish Tagging Panels is the Team Management tools. These tools allow for a database of team/player names to be kept so that they can be selected when analysing specific games. Team and individual player data are added to the database using the Team Manager

34

tool. When the relevant individual players have been selected from the Team Manager list prior to initial tagging, these players' names will appear in the Team Group Box linked to the Team Manager. These player names can be set up to either represent Events, Continuous Events, Keywords or Persistent Keywords.

All of the tools mentioned can be used within the Tagging Panel in a direct linear fashion or by using the layout tools organised to make it more ergonomic and efficient for the tagging process. There are two types of layout tools; a Group Box and a Tab Group Box. These layout tools perform two functions: first they allow users to organise the layout of their Tagging Panel by grouping similar buttons together; second, they can provide the categories within which these buttons are grouped.

### Triggers/reset

To allow the creation of a more ergonomic Tagging Panel design, users can control the flow of their tagging panel by setting up triggers within button properties to allow the automatic activation or deactivation of other relevant tagging panel items, i.e. this can be used between an event and a stacked tab group box containing multiple keyword buttons. Similarly to this there is an option to reset category properties to deactivate continuous or persistent buttons, i.e. if possession is being tagged, events such as shot on goal can be made to reset all buttons with player as a category as no player will have possession. Care must be taken with the spelling of these categories and buttons as they must match with exact spelling and spacing.

When administered in a Tagging Panel, these buttons provide the data to fill the 'Name' column of the Events List and allow further data to be added. Each time an event is recorded, the standard information that is noted alongside it is the time it occurred (noted in the Position column) and the duration of the event (in the Duration column). In order to see more data regarding these events, such as the keywords, categories need to be set up using the Tagging Panel to group together the event and keyword. Figure 2.5 is an example of an Events List.

To interrogate the data collected, Tables and Keywords can be used. These can normally be found to the left of the Events List frame. Keywords provide a frequency list of the number of times each keyword

| # | Name | Position | Duration | Game Set Pieces | Shot Outcome |
|---|------|----------|----------|-----------------|--------------|
| 1 | Corner | 13 sec | 6 sec | | |
| 2 | Shot | 18 sec | 7 sec | Shot | Blocked |

Figure 2.5 Dartfish Events List with category titles

has been attributed to an event while the Tables section allows for a more detailed interrogation of the variables collected, by cross tabulating the Category titles from the tagging panels. This cross-tabulated data can be presented in either a frequency of events format, a percentage of the total number, or as duration of the events. Users can add extra categories to drill deeper into the data by adding column or row labels. These data can be exported as a table by right clicking the table and selecting Export Table and then saving as a comma separated file. The data from the Events List can also be exported and processed as a spreadsheet in Excel. Chapter 3 will provide some details about the different types of formulae that can be applied to this type of data.

Creation of interactive video feedback is also possible from the table data within Dartfish by selecting the values from the cross-tabulated categories. This filters the Events List providing the relevant clips selected from the table. These clips can then be added to the Storyboard for annotation and animation for the creation of feedback videos.

## SUMMARY

Commercial video analysis packages are generic, allowing them to be used with any game sport. Users create metadata to represent the sport-specific system to be implemented in the package. The main analysis feature of all of the packages is the ability to cross-tabulate variables allowing frequencies to be displayed. Criteria can be established allowing users to select video sequences representing aspects of the game requiring attention. These video sequences can be viewed interactively within the packages or included within highlights movies that can be created. The chronologically ordered list of match events can be exported for further analysis in general purpose packages such as Microsoft Excel.

# CHAPTER 3

## MICROSOFT EXCEL

### INTRODUCTION

Microsoft Excel is a spreadsheet application developed by Microsoft, available for both Microsoft Windows and Apple Mac operating systems. It is worth noting that not all the functions and features that are commonly found in the Windows version are in the Mac Excel version. The software allows for the organising of and formatting of data arranged in rows and columns that can be manipulated by mathematical formulae and functions to perform a number of basic and more complex calculations. It also allows for the creation of tables and graphs to visually represent data.

This chapter discusses the most useful features of Excel for processing sports performance data. The chapter does not intend to cover all of the features that Excel has to offer, but it highlights how data from performance analysis packages can be processed and manipulated. Excel has a wealth of facilities and functions and this chapter could only cover a fraction of them. The use of basic arithmetic, logical operators, text processing and conditional functions are all covered. Excel allows data and the functions that process them to be included on the same worksheet and spreadsheets can be made up of a series of worksheets. Pivot tables are very useful in performance analysis and can allow rapid processing of Event Lists exported from commercial packages. Table lookup features, absolute, relative and indirect addressing are all covered. Sorting, filtering, producing charts and protecting worksheets are also covered. The chapter uses example worksheets found on the Routledge website tab for this textbook. These worksheets are found in the spreadsheet file 'Data Analysis in Sport.xls' unless specifically stated otherwise.

## CREATING AND OPENING SPREADSHEETS

### Creating a spreadsheet

Statistics packages, such as SPSS, separate data from the resulting analysis output and also use columns for variables and rows for cases (units of analysis). Microsoft Excel offers much greater flexibility in that rows or columns could be used to represent variables or cases. The data for a particular case could be entered into several rows (or columns). Users have the option to use one or several worksheets within the package to represent the data. One strategy is to include different stages of data processing on different worksheets. The functions that process data and evaluate intermediate or final results can be included on the same worksheets as the data. Charts can also be included on the same worksheets as the data or presented on their own sheets. Therefore, those developing spreadsheets in Excel should plan how their spreadsheets are going to store and process data and present resulting information. Once this is done, a new spreadsheet can be opened and data can be entered into it. This task typically happens when data have been recorded on manual notation forms or other sources that cannot be loaded directly into Excel.

### Data opening

Most sports performance analysis packages allow for data collected to be exported in a format that Excel can interpret. This is sometimes done as an Excel file but other packages export data as a comma-separated values (.csv) file. The CSV format allows the storing of tabular-based data in plain-text form. To open this data file in Excel, users need to follow the steps on the Text Import Wizard. This allows Excel to identify the characters that have been used to separate the data into different columns. Delimited is selected as an option in Step 1 as shown in Figure 3.1. Figure 3.2 shows Step 2 where a Delimiter used in the plain text file, such as comma, tab or spaces, is selected. For example, Dartfish exports an Events List using a Tab delimiter. The appropriate delimiter can be easily identified by viewing the Data Preview when the relevant delimiters are selected. As long as the data are organised as expected within the columns displayed in the preview area, then the correct Delimiter has been selected. Step 3 allows users to tell Excel how to format the data in each column. This is illustrated in Figure 3.3. Excel uses the General

38

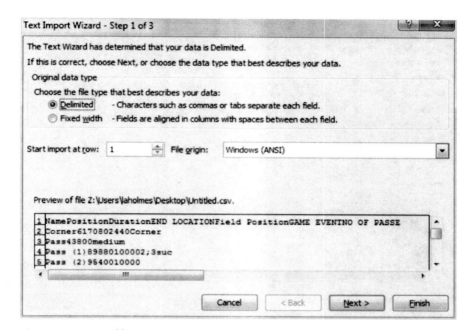

Figure 3.1 CSV file input: step 1

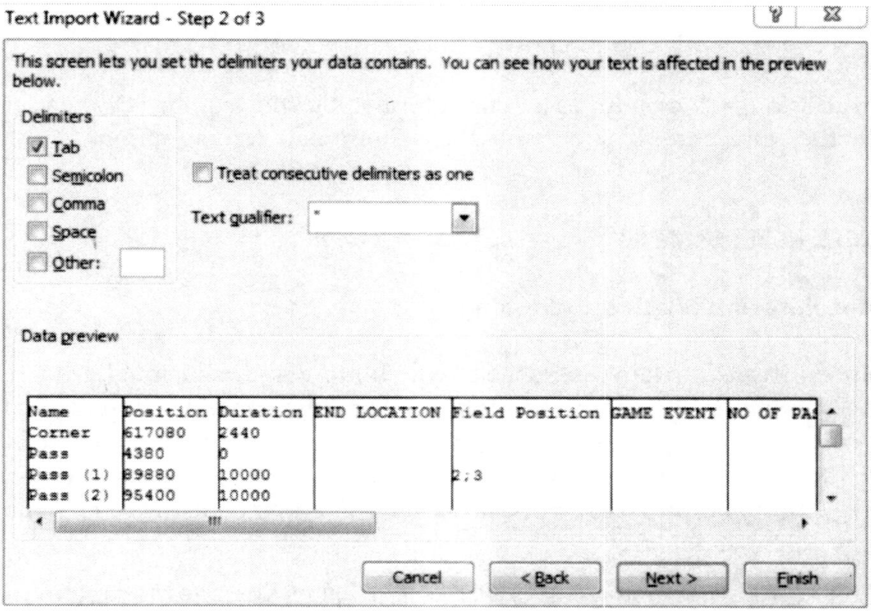

Figure 3.2 CSV file input: step 2

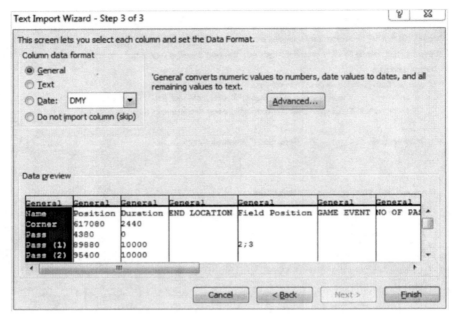

Figure 3.3 CSV file input: step 3

format for each column as a default format, but this can be adjusted for each column individually using the Column data format options.

## CELL REFERENCING

### Absolute and relative addressing

Spreadsheets contain worksheets, which are two-dimensional grids of cells. Some cells contain data while other cells contain functions and expressions that process data. Therefore, it is essential to be able to refer to the locations of data as well as the results evaluated by functions and expressions. Most Excel worksheets refer to columns using letters and rows using numbers.

The use of cell referencing is very useful when it comes to creating a spreadsheet into which you can paste your raw data and quickly produce outputs using pre-programmed calculations. Controlling the order of the columns and rows of data from analysis software packages (see Chapter 2) enables spreadsheets to be set up that will automatically complete further calculations upon a 'data dump'. This also allows dashboard style reports representing relevant data to be completed (see Chapter 4).

Cell referencing works by including the location of the cells that you want to use, as opposed to the exact data values that are currently displayed there; the values can change as data they use change. Consider the first cell in a work sheet, A1, which is located at the top left hand corner of the worksheet. Any formula including a reference to the cell A1, will use the data currently displayed in A1. When the data value in A1 changes, the calculations are redone in any cells referring to A1 and the values that they display will change accordingly.

Table 3.1 shows four different ways of addressing the cell B2. The row, column or both the row and column where a cell is located can be fixed within a formula using absolute references. This is done using the '$' symbol before the column and/or row of interest. This is important to remember when pasting cells containing formulae into other cell locations. Consider the cell F2 containing a formula that refers to B2 as a relative reference (without using the '$' symbol). If the formula in F2 is pasted into further cells in column F (say F3, F4 and F5), then the new copies of the formula will reference the cells in column B in the same rows (specifically B3, B4 and B5). Similarly, if the formula in F2 is pasted into further cells in row 2 (say G2, H2 and I2), then the new copies of the formula will reference the cells in row 2 that are five cells to the left of their locations (specifically C2, D2 and E2). In other words, a relative reference to B2 within the cell F2 is referring to the cell that is five cells to the left. If, when pasting, we wanted formulae to continue to refer to the specific cell B2 rather than making relative references, we would use $B$2.

Table 3.1 **Cell referencing**

| Reference formula | Description |
| --- | --- |
| B2 | Relative cell reference |
| $B2 | Absolute column reference |
| B$2 | Absolute row reference |
| $B$2 | Absolute column and row reference |

41

Figure 3.4 gives an example of the combined use of relative and absolute addressing. The number of passes made by four national teams are stored in the cells B2 to E2 with the cell G2 showing the total number of passes. When the cells B4 to E4 are formatted to show percentages, the percentage of passes played by each national team can be displayed without having to multiply the fraction by 100. Consider the percentage of all passes that were made by Wales. The cell B4 refers to B2 so that when it is pasted into C4 to E4, these cells will make relative reference to the cells that are two cells above them (C2 to E2). The cell B4 uses the '$' sign in the formula to keep the cell reference referring to the same column. So that when you copy the cell formula across to other columns for the calculation of percentages for England, Scotland and Ireland it still refers to column G. With the '$' being placed just in front of the column letter, this fixes the reference to the column, but will still allow it to change the row number it refers to.

When compiling formulae into the formula bar, you can use the keyboard shortcut of F4 (Windows) or CMD+T (Mac) to toggle between the specific cell referencing options.

Some functions use multiple values and multiple cells, which can be expressed as specific cells separated by commas (for example 'B2, E2' refers to the two cells B2 and E2) or a range of cells using colons (for example 'B2:E2' refers to the four cells B2, C2, D2 and E2). The range of cells referred to using the colon can be a two dimensional array of cells, for example B2:E5 refers to a 4 × 4 array of cells. Arrays of cells can be referred to relatively or absolutely the same way as single cells can be. It is also possible to reference cells within other worksheets by appending the name of the worksheet in the formula followed by an exclamation mark '!' to the start of the cell reference. For example, 'Edit_List!C2' refers to the cell C2 in the worksheet 'Edit_List' while 'Table!B2' refers to the cell B2 within the worksheet 'Table'. This is very helpful, when users

|  | A | B | C | D | E | F | G |
|---|---|---|---|---|---|---|---|
| 1 |  | Wales | England | Scotland | Ireland |  | Total |
| 2 | Passes | 66 | 52 | 44 | 33 |  | 195 |
| 3 |  |  |  |  |  |  |  |
| 4 | Percentage | =B2/$G2 | =C2/$G2 | =D2/$G2 | =E2/$G2 |  |  |

Figure 3.4 Formula using Cell Referencing

42

want to have one worksheet to 'dump' from external sources without negatively impacting on the cell references and calculations that have already been created to perform subsequent calculations. This enables a swift turnaround of data representation mid and post analysis (see the 'Edit_List' and 'Game counts' worksheets).

## The INDIRECT function

The INDRECT function is a useful tool that allows the creation of references to cells and ranges from contents contained within other cells, rather than the exact reference in the formula. INDIRECT will turn any string information into an exact reference, so that references to cells can be constructed from a combination of string constants and values contained within other cells.

## Named ranges

Organising and using spreadsheets that contain numerous columns of data can be a daunting task, but it is something that every analyst needs to do on a regular basis. Creating formulae that reference data already arranged in columns and more likely with column headings can be easier to manage if named ranges are utilised. Normal cell referencing would refer to the specific cells within the range that contains the data by relative row and column information. Using named ranges eliminates the need for specific row and column-based references, instead replacing these with individual names. You can create defined named ranges to represent cells, ranges of cells, formulas, constant values or tables. These names then indicate the relative positioning of the data. Since named ranges do not change when a formula is copied to other cells, this provides an alternative to using absolute cell references in functions and formulae. This also allows users to set up ranges to allow extra data to be added at a later stage. An example of this is found in the 'Premier League Match Results' worksheet. To set up named ranges in the Windows version of Excel use **Formulas → Define Name**. On the Mac version of Excel this is done using **Insert → Name → Define**. Users will need to input a name to call the range and provide the range of cell references to which it refers. If cells where there is not currently data are included, when you use these named ranges in formulae, the error checking routines will indicate an error. Error Checking within Excel Options (Windows) or Excel Preferences (Mac) allows error reporting to be turned off when a formula refers to an empty cell.

## PROCESSING NUMERICAL DATA

### Time data transformations

Time-based data that are exported from analysis packages do not necessarily conform to the formats that Excel recognises. In order to be able to conduct some calculations using these data, they must first be transformed. Dartfish time-based data actually includes the individual frame numbers of the video it is referencing. Therefore, the 'Position' column of the exported data contains values like 482880. There are two things that need to be done to such data as shown in Figure 3.5. Initially the values need to be recalculated using the formula in cell L2.

The formula is a basic calculation that uses the data in cell 'B2' and then performs a division calculation thereafter, providing the value of 0.002249074. Second, by formatting this value as a custom time format (hh:mm:ss.00), we will have a usable time format that Excel will recognise, and with which be able to perform many various calculations.

SportsCode data export via the Edit List, produces time-based data, that on initial viewing appear to be actual time-based data. On closer inspection, however, there is a minor anomaly where the last digits in a value represent the milliseconds of the time data and are separated from the seconds by a colon. The colon should really be a period. With the data in this format, Excel does not recognise it as time based data, but as a

| | A | B | .... | L |
|---|---|---|---|---|
| 1 | | Position | | Position |
| 2 | | 194320 | | =B2/1000/60/60/24 |
| . | | . | | . |
| . | | . | | . |
| 30 | | 853600 | | =B30/1000/60/60/24 |

Figure 3.5 Time transformation from Dartfish data export

44

|   | A | B | C |
|---|---|---|---|
| 1 | Start time | | START TIME |
| 2 | 00:00:02:62 | ..... | =TIMEVALUE(SUBSTITUTE(A2,":",".",3)) |
| . | . | | . |
| . | . | | . |
| 30 | 00:00:24:73 | | =TIMEVALUE(SUBSTITUTE(A30,":",".",3)) |

Figure 3.6 Time transformation from SportsCode data export

text string. Therefore, mathematical calculations cannot use the data in their current form. The formula in Figure 3.6 uses the SUBSTITUTE function to replace the colon with a period and the TIMEVALUE function converts the text string into an integer-based time value. This value can be formatted using the same custom time format (hh:mm:ss.00) as with Dartfish explained above. Now that the time is in a recognisable format for Excel, any calculations necessary can be made with reference to those specific cells.

## Basic mathematical formulae

All formulae in Excel start with an equal sign (=). Following this are the elements to be calculated separated by the numerical, logical or text processing operators. Excel calculates formulae by applying operators in descending order of operator precedence (or priority order), applying operators of the same precedence from left to right. Arithmetic operators include addition (+), subtraction (−), multiplication (*), division (/) and power (^). The order that calculations are undertaken in can be referred to as the 'BODMAS' order, which is shown in Table 3.2.

Table 3.2 BODMAS order of operations in formulae

| Operator | Description |
|---|---|
| B | Brackets |
| O | Orders (powers and square roots) |
| DM | Division and Multiplication (left-to-right) |
| AS | Addition and Subtraction (left-to-right) |

Consider two cells, B2 and B3, that are currently evaluated to 3 and 4 respectively. The following expression is evaluated to 3.5.

=B2/(B3−1) * SQRT(B3)+2*B2/B3

This is because the '(B3−1)' is evaluated first as brackets have the highest priority. This reduced the expression to:

=B2/3 * SQRT(B3)+2*B2/B3

The function call 'SQRT(B3)' is the square root of 4 which is 2, reducing the expression to:

=B2/3 * 2 + 2*B2/B3

The '*' and '/' operators are then evaluated from left to right reducing the expression to:

=2+1.5

Any numerical constants, values, variables (cell references) and function calls can be formed into an expression contained within a cell using these arithmetic operators. Excel provides different classes of functions that produce numerical mathematical, statistical, trigonometric and financial calculations. The 'SQRT' function is one of these functions and readers are encouraged to browse the different types of function available in Excel. The Insert Function popup window gives excellent information on the purpose of each function and the number and type of arguments used.

**Viewing Formulae**

This chapter has shown formulae within cells as well as values that these formulae produce. Usually we view the latter with the formulae in the current cell viewable in a function preview area of the Excel interface. However, there are occasions where viewing functions is more beneficial than viewing the values they currently yield. One example of this is to assist in the error checking process of formulae. It is helpful to be able to see the formulae all interacting together. By pressing CTRL+` you can

# 46

toggle between displaying the actual values and the formulas contained. This does not change the state of the cells.

## CONDITIONAL FORMULAE

### The IF function

The 'IF' function allows us to evaluate expressions based on the truth of conditional tests. The 'IF' function can be used with or without an alternative expression to be evaluated if the condition is False. The first form is illustrated in the following example:

=IF(B2 > 0, A2 / B2)

This avoids a division by zero error by only evaluating A2/B2 if B2 is greater than zero. Where B2 is zero or less, this 'IF' function will evaluate to False. The following is an example of the second way the 'IF' statement can be used.

=IF(B2 >= 40, "Pass", "Fail")

The cell B2 could contain an examination result and the 'IF' function evaluates to a character string that indicates whether the exam has been passed or not. Table 3.3 shows the main comparison operators that can be used within the conditions of 'IF' functions.

The example in Figure 3.7 queries the values found in column B against column D, returning values from A or E. If the score found in the cell in column B is greater than the score in the cell in column E, it will return

Table 3.3 Comparison operators

| Comparison operator | Meaning (example) |
|---|---|
| = (Equal sign) | Equal to (A1=B1) |
| > (Greater than sign) | Greater than (A1>B1) |
| < (Less than sign) | Less than (A1<B1) |
| >= (Greater than or equal to sign) | Greater than or equal to (A1>=B1) |
| <= (Less than or equal to sign) | Less than or equal to (A1<=B1) |
| <> (Not equal to sign) | Not equal to (A1<>B1) |

| | A | B | C | D | E | F | G |
|---|---|---|---|---|---|---|---|
| 1 | **HOME** | | | | **AWAY** | | **WINNER** |
| 2 | Liverpool | 5 | - | 1 | Arsenal | | =IF(B2>D2,A2,E2) |
| 3 | Aston Villa | 0 | - | 2 | West Ham | | =IF(B3>D3,A3,E3) |
| 4 | Chelsea | 3 | - | 0 | Newcastle | | =IF(B4>D4,A4,E4) |
| 5 | Crystal Palace | 3 | - | 1 | West Brom | | =IF(B5>D5,A5,E5) |

Figure 3.7 Application of the 'IF' function

the cell value in column A. If this condition is found to be False, then it will return value in column E. Therefore, the 'IF' function will report the team with the greatest number of goals scored.

'IF' functions can be used within expressions and can also be used within other 'IF' functions. Once 'IF' statements are nested beyond a depth of three levels they are difficult to maintain. When using nested 'IF' functions, the inner 'IF' function could be the expression used if the outer condition is True or if it is False. When the inner 'IF' function is evaluated when the outer condition is False, it becomes the 'else do this' part for the first 'IF' function. By using nested 'IF' functions and different comparisons, the example in Figure 3.8 reports the name of the winning team if there is a winner, if not it will report 'DRAW'. Note how the subsequent 'IF' statements provide the 'else do this' element of the function.

'IF' functions could be nested to evaluate some expression if two conditions are true. However, this would be better achieved using a single 'IF' function where a single condition uses an 'AND' operator to combine the two Boolean conditions. Boolean conditions can be combined using logical operators; 'AND' and 'OR' with 'NOT' being used with a single condition where appropriate. These are summarised in Table 3.4. The 'Game Counts' worksheet references data from an exported Edit List and

| | A | B | C | D | E | F | G |
|---|---|---|---|---|---|---|---|
| 1 | **HOME** | | | | **AWAY** | | **WINNER** |
| 2 | Cardiff | 0 | - | 0 | Aston Villa | | =IF(B2>D2,A2,IF(B2<D2,E2, "DRAW")) |
| 3 | Hull | 0 | - | 1 | Southampton | | =IF(B3>D3,A3,IF(B3<D3,E3, "DRAW")) |
| 4 | West Ham | 2 | - | 0 | Norwich | | =IF(B4>D4,A4,IF(B4<D4,E4, "DRAW")) |
| 5 | West Brom | 1 | - | 1 | Chelsea | | =IF(B5>D5,A5,IF(B5<D5,E5, "DRAW")) |

Figure 3.8 Application of nested IF functions

48

**Table 3.4** Logical operators descriptors

| Logical operator | Meaning (example) |
| --- | --- |
| AND | =AND(first condition, second condition, ... etc.) |
| OR | =OR(first condition, second condition, ... etc.) |
| NOT | =NOT(condition) |

interrogates the data for occurrences that match based on two criteria by combining the 'IF' and 'AND' functions into one formula and returning a value based on the findings.

**COUNT and COUNTIF**

The COUNT group of functions can be used to further process data collected. COUNT by itself is a fairly easy function that just provides the total number of numerical values in a given range of cells. The COUNTIF function is a decidedly more powerful function and used extensively within the 'Premier League Summary' worksheet. The COUNTIF function counts the number of occurrences within a range of cells where the data meet the criterion specified.

COUNTIFS allows for multiple criteria to be set within the formula and counts the number of times all these criteria are met. We can use up to 127 range/criteria within this function. As with all formulae, each criterion is tested one cell at a time, if these are met in the first cell, then the count increases by 1, if the second cell satisfies the criteria, the count increases by 1 again, until all cells within the range have been tested.

In the 'Premier League Summary' worksheet, named ranges have been set to allow easier references to individual column data. For example, the formula in cell K2 tests the cells associated within the range named 'Result', to see if it matches the contents of cell K1 and then test cells within the range 'Won' for contents of J2. Each time these criteria are met, it counts their occurrence and returns the total number in the cell. The following function allows the spreadsheet to calculate the number of times a team has Won, Lost or Drawn a game. Figure 3.9 illustrates this using columns F to G to show results and columns J and K to show the number of home wins for the teams. Note the use of the cell reference to provide the information for the criteria, as opposed to a constant value.

=COUNTIFS(Result,K$1,Won,$J2)

| ... | F | G | H | I | J | K |
|---|---|---|---|---|---|---|
| 1 | Result | Won | Lost | | SUMMARY | HOME WIN |
| 2 | AWAY WIN | Aston Villa | Arsenal | | Arsenal | =COUNTIFS(Result,K$1,Won,$J2) |
| 3 | HOME WIN | Liverpool | Stoke | | Aston Villa | 4 |
| 4 | DRAW | Norwich | Everton | | Cardiff | 5 |
| 5 | AWAY WIN | Fulham | Sunderland | | Chelsea | 13 |
| 6 | AWAY WIN | Man United | Swansea | | | |

Figure 3.9 Application of COUNTIFS function

## TEXT PROCESSING

### The Slam Tracker example

On some occasions there may need to be several steps to the data handling and preparation before you can get it to a useable state to undertake further calculations. This is especially the case if there is lots of text-based information, for example from IBM Slam Tracker website. The 'slamtracker.xls' spreadsheet processes Slam Tracker data from the US Open through several stages shown on five separate worksheets within the file.

Slam Tracker data include details of each point played. The points are shown in reverse order with point details in a row and then the game score as a result of the point. For example, Figure 3.10 is a section of data copied and pasted from the 2013 US Open men's singles final. Rafael Nadal lost the first point making it 15–0 (last two rows of Figure 3.10 because the data are in reverse order) which tells us that Novak Djokovic was serving in the first game. There were 223 points in the match.

We wish to produce a list of points in the correct order that contains the following details:

Column A: Point number
Column B: Point details as expressed in Slamtracker
Column C: Game score after the point
Column D: Server
Column E: Player ending the point
Column F: Outcome with respect to the player ending the point (W or L)
Column G: Outcome with respect to the serving player (W or L)

# 50

| | |
|---|---|
| 0-0 | Game score after last point |
| N. Djokovic loses the match with a forehand unforced error. | Last point |
| 15-40 | |
| N. Djokovic loses the point with a forehand forced error. | |
| 15-30 | |
| R. Nadal wins the point with a forehand winner. | |
| . <br> . <br> . | |
| 30-15 | |
| R. Nadal loses the point with a backhand unforced error. | |
| 15-15 | |
| N. Djokovic loses the point with a backhand volley forced error. | |
| 15-0 | Game score after first point |
| R. Nadal loses the point with a forehand forced error. | First point |

Figure 3.10 Slam Tracker tennis data pasted into Excel

The following steps are used to arrange the data into the required format.

## 1. Copy points from Slam Tracker

Copy the point list from Slam Tracker and paste into Excel. This is the 'As Pasted' worksheet. Note the points are in reverse order and there are 2 rows per point; one for the point score after the point and one for the text description of the point.

## 2. Arrange points into order

Copy the data into the third column of a new sheet; see the 'Working 1' worksheet. In cells A1 and A2 type '1' and '1' to signify this is the first point shown (it's actually the last point). In cell B1 type 'Score' and in cell B2 type 'Point'. Now to save ourselves a lot of typing, type '=A1+1' in the cell A3. This is basically adding 1 to the point number. Now type '=B1' in the cell B3. This means that the contents of column B are the same as what we see two rows earlier ('Score' or 'Point'). Now select A3:B3 and paste all the way down for the remainder of columns A and B.

Now copy all of the information in columns A, B and C and select these same cells but use **Paste-Values** to only store the values in the cells, over-writing the functions that were there. This is important because we are about to sort the data and we need the values to be unaltered. Now sort columns A, B and C on column B (ordered A to Z) and then add a level to then sort by column A (sorted largest to smallest to get the points in the correct order). We now have all of the point details followed by all of the point scores. Cut the point scores and paste them into the cells D2:D223 so that they are beside the point details for the correct points.

We can now delete the rows after row 223. We can also delete column B; we know the rows contain point details. The point numbers are in the reverse order 223, 222, 221, …, 1 but the point details are in the right order. So just select column A only. Sort this column on column A (small-est to largest). Excel will query why you are only sorting a single column. Just confirm that this is what you want to do. Now the points are in the correct order and numbered 1, 2, 3,…, 223. We can insert a row of head-ings 'Point No', 'Details' and 'Score After' in row 1. We are now left with what we see in the sheet 'Working 2'.

### 3. Determine who served

Look for the first ace (use the find facility). It is point 6 where N. Djokovic serves an ace. We can easily work out from this that N. Djokovic served first. Even if the first ace was much later, we could work out who served first in the first game based on the scores of 0–0, which signify the end of games. Insert a new heading 'Server' into the cell D1. Type 'N. Djokovic' into cell D2 to signify that he served in the first point. Now we need to populate the rest of column D by assuming the serving player is the same as in the previous point unless the score at the end of the previ-ous point was 0–0. This is done using the following nested 'IF' function, which we type into cell D3:

=IF(C2= "0–0", IF(D2= "N. Djokovic", "R. Nadal", "N. Djokovic"), D2)

This asks if the score in the previous point was '0–0'. If it was we need to change the server using the inner 'IF' function, otherwise we simply use the server in the previous point who is specified in cell D2. If this is a change of games, the inner 'IF' function simply asks if the server in the previous point was N. Djokovic. If it was then the server in the next point is R. Nadal, otherwise it is N. Djokovic. Copy this function in cell D3 and paste into the cells D3:D224. This results in what we see in the worksheet 'Server'.

At this point we should check the match score on the official tournament website (2013.usopen.org) to make sure there were no tiebreakers. In this case, the score was 6–2, 3–6, 6–4, 6–1. If the match had involved tiebreakers, we would need to copy the server information, pasting these values over the functions and then locate the tiebreaker (the point scores are different for tiebreakers; they use 0, 1, 2, … instead of 0, 15, 30, …) and manually key in the serving player, making sure they alternate after every odd point of the tiebreaker. Note the player serving first in the tiebreaker is different to the player who served first in the previous game. Also, the player who serves in the first game of any set after a tiebreaker is the same player who served in the game before the tiebreaker.

### 4. Determine the player whose action (whether ace, double fault, winner or error) ended the point

This next step is illustrated in column E of the worksheet 'Player'. Consider the text 'R. Nadal loses …' The player's name ends with a space character (' '). This is the second space in the text because there is a space between the player's initial and surname. We can find the location of this second space by using the FIND function in Excel as follows (assuming we do this in E2 referring to data in row 2):

=FIND(" ", B2, 4)

This looks for a space in the text detail for the point starting at character 4 which is after the first space. In this case the value is 9. So the name 'R. Nadal' is obtained from the left-most 8 characters of the cell B2. We cannot use LEFT(B2, 8) because two different players are involved in the match. So we use the 'FIND' function within the 'LEFT' function in cell E2 as follows:

=LEFT(B2, FIND(" " , B2, 4)–1)

## 5. Determining the outcome of the point and the point winner

This next step is illustrated in columns F and G of the 'Player' worksheet. First, column F deals with the player whose action ended the point. The point details consist of a player's name and then the word 'wins' or 'loses'. This word exists between the second and third spaces so we could write a function to determine the word ('wins' or 'loses'). However, we only need the first letter to distinguish the point outcome for the player whose action ended the point. We can use the same function FIND(" ", B2, 4) to determine the location of the last space before the 'w' or 'l'. The MID function in Excel evaluates to a string of characters in the middle of some existing string of characters. So if B2 contains the text 'R. Nadal loses ...' then MID(B2, 10, 1) gives us the 1 character starting at the 10th character in the string which is 'l'. Once again we wish to use this with both players so we use FIND to locate the character before 'loses' as follows in cell F2:

=MID(B2, FIND(" ", B2, 4) +1 ,1)

Column G deals with the serving player, determining whether they won or lost the point. If the serving player is the same player as the player who ended the point then we can use that player's outcome, otherwise we need to use the opposite outcome. This is achieved in the cell G2 using a nested 'IF' function. The serving player and player whose action ended the point are found in cells D2 and E2 respectively. We ask if these two players are the same and if they are then the outcome with respect to the serving player is taken from cell F2 because it is the same as that of the player who ended the point. If this is not the case, then the outcome for the server is opposite to that in F2. So if F2 contains 'w' then the inner 'IF' function evaluates to 'l' otherwise it evaluates to 'w'. The nested 'IF' statement in G2 is, therefore, as follows:

=IF(D2=E2, F2, IF(F2= "w", "l", "w"))

## TABLE LOOKUP FUNCTIONS

### LOOKUP functions

Consider the worksheet 'Table'. This contains a table of 33 rows; one row of headings and then 32 rows of data as shown in Figure 3.11.

# 54

|  | A | B | C |
|---|---|---|---|
| 1 | Team | Ranking points | Distance to Brasilia |
| 2 | Algeria | 792 | 7914 |
| 3 | Argentina | 1251 | 2304 |
| 4 | Australia | 571 | 14058 |
| 5 | Belgium | 1098 | 8967 |
| 6 | Bosnia | 899 | 9420 |
| 7 | Brazil | 1102 | 0 |
| 8 | Cameroon | 616 | 6715 |
| 9 | Chile | 1005 | 3002 |
| 10 | Columbia | 1200 | 3669 |
| 11 | Costa Rica | 743 | 4903 |
| 12 | Croatia | 971 | 9361 |
| 13 | Ecuador | 852 | 3782 |
| 14 | England | 1041 | 8781 |
| 15 | France | 893 | 8713 |
| 16 | Germany | 1318 | 9579 |
| 17 | Ghana | 851 | 5772 |
| 18 | Greece | 1055 | 9552 |
| 19 | Holland | 1106 | 9104 |
| 20 | Honduras | 692 | 5446 |
| 21 | Iran | 727 | 11865 |
| 22 | Italy | 1120 | 8906 |
| 23 | Ivory Coast | 912 | 5326 |
| 24 | Japan | 641 | 17683 |
| 25 | Korea | 581 | 17548 |
| 26 | Mexico | 892 | 6835 |
| 27 | Nigeria | 701 | 6139 |
| 28 | Portugal | 1172 | 7270 |
| 29 | Russia | 870 | 11175 |
| 30 | Spain | 1507 | 7728 |
| 31 | Switzerland | 1113 | 8876 |
| 32 | Uruguay | 1132 | 2257 |
| 33 | USA | 1019 | 6778 |

Figure 3.11 Information on teams contesting the 2014 FIFA World Cup

In the sheet, 'Table Look Up' we use the VLOOKUP function to determine the FIFA World ranking points and distance to Brasilia for England and Italy. This is shown in Figure 3.12. Consider the cell B2. The vertical lookup function here looks up the current value of A2 (England) in the left most column of the array A$2:A$33 in the sheet 'Table'. This determines the row (14) where the required value will be found. The third argument of the function specified the column that contains the value of interest, in this case the second column of the array (which is

|   | A | B | C |
|---|---|---|---|
| 1 | Team | Ranking Points | Distance to Brasilia |
| 2 | England | =VLOOKUP(A2,Table!A$2:C$33,2,False) | =VLOOKUP(A2,Table!A$2:C$33,3,False) |
| 3 | Italy | =VLOOKUP(A3,Table!A$2:C$33,2,False) | =VLOOKUP(A3,Table!A$2:C$33,3,False) |

Figure 3.12 Use of the VLOOKUP function

column B). If the last argument was 'True' then the VLOOKUP function would look for the closest matching value to 'England' where the values are sorted in ascending order. In this case, the final argument is 'False' and so VLOOKUP looks for an exact match. The value in the cell B14 of the sheet 'Table' is 1041 and so this value will be displayed in cell B2 of the 'Table Look Up' sheet. HLOOKUP is similar to VLOOKUP except it searches for the given value in row 1 and looks up a corresponding value in a specified row rather than column.

The LOOKUP functions return a value from either one row or one column range for a value, and then returns a value from the same position in a second row or column range. You can perform these LOOKUP functions either vertically (VLOOKUP) or horizontally (HLOOKUP). There is a more general 'LOOKUP' function that requires three arguments (the results vector is optional) as follows:

=LOOKUP(specific value to lookup, lookup range of one row/column, result vector)

### INDEX and MATCH functions

INDEX and MATCH are two members of the LOOKUP function group. The basic INDEX function returns a value based on an array or column and row number.

=INDEX(array, row_num/col_num)

MATCH searches a range of cells for a specified value and then returns the relative position of the value within the range.

=MATCH(lookup_value, lookup_array, [match_type])

56

Combining INDEX and MATCH functions is a powerful way of looking up data within tables. MATCH can provide the value for the row_num argument within the INDEX function.

Although this function combination performs similar lookups to a VLOOKUP, they are actually simpler and easier to set up. A VLOOKUP requires the whole array table to be selected, whilst the INDEX MATCH function combination just needs the lookup column and the return column. So, when we are working with large amounts of data, which we may well be, this will be a simpler process.

The worksheet 'PIVOT FTHG' uses the formulae in Figure 3.13 to report the Highest Goal scoring team and Lowest Goal scoring team. Another added reason for using INDEX and MATCH lookup functions over VLOOKUP is the fact that they can be set up to perform dynamically.

## PIVOT TABLES

Pivot tables allow us to more easily summarise and analyse large volumes of data. They are a great tool for sorting, tabulating and summarising the data collected. We can control how the data are tabulated and the summaries are presented using sums, frequencies or averages (means). Many analysts shy away from using them, thinking they are too hard. However, the benefits of using pivot tables with Event Lists exported from video analysis packages makes it well worth analysts' time learning how to use them. In essence we are comparing rows and columns of data, and the pivot table builder allows us to select which data variables to place in rows and columns.

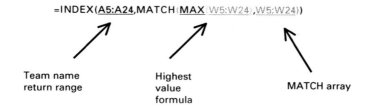

Figure 3.13 Combined use of the INDEX and MATCH functions

The 'possession_events.xls' spreadsheet file is an example of using pivot tables to summarise data exported from the Focus X2 package. The data are seen in the 'Raw' worksheet where we select all 9 columns and use **Insert → Pivot Table** electing to store the pivot table in a new worksheet that we have called 'Pivot'. In the 'Pivot Field List' (Figure 3.14) drag and drop 'Type' into the 'Row Labels' and 'Outcome' into 'Column Labels'. Then drag and drop 'Duration' into the 'Values'. We want to show the average duration of possessions for each type of outcome. This is done by clicking on the arrow at the right hand side of 'Duration' in the values box and select 'Value Field Settings' and then selecting 'AVERAGE' from the 'Summarizes Values By' list (see Figure 3.15). The resulting pivot table is shown in Figure 3.16.

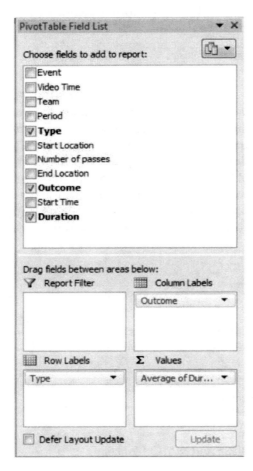

Figure 3.14 The Pivot Table Builder interface

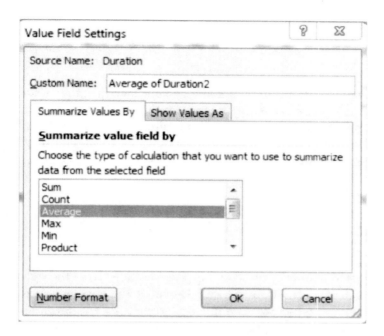

Figure 3.15 Changing value field setting in a pivot table to see the mean value

| Average of Duration2 | Column Labels | | | | | | | | |
|---|---|---|---|---|---|---|---|---|---|
| Row Labels | Ball out of play | Free conceded | Goal | Interception | Shot off target | Shot on target | Tackled | (blank) | Grand Total |
| Corner | | 4.88 | | 8.47 | | | 7.64 | | 7.72 |
| Free kick | 7.911111111 | 8.59 | | 8.22 | 6.8 | 6.2 | 6.985714286 | | 7.757692308 |
| Interception | 7.8575 | 7.173333333 | 10.76 | 7.49037037 | 6.34 | | 7.749333333 | | 7.5604 |
| Kick off | | | | 11.64 | | | | 8.64 | 10.14 |
| Tackle | 7.4775 | 7.9 | | 7.388148148 | | 10.44 | 7.176842105 | | 7.487272727 |
| Throw in | 7 | 7.993333333 | | 6.687058824 | | | 6.578181818 | | 6.9 |
| (blank) | | | | | | | | | |
| Grand Total | 7.62893617 | 7.550204082 | 10.76 | 7.568979592 | 6.493333333 | 7.613333333 | 7.310649351 | | 7.504604317 |

Figure 3.16 Pivot table showing the mean duration of each possession type and each outcome

If readers are doing this in Excel for Mac, Pivot Table can be found in the Data tab rather than the Insert tab. Select the variables to be tabulated using the 'Pivot Table Builder' and adjust the individual value settings by clicking on the information 'i' icon.

# FORMATTING

## Formatting cells

Earlier in this chapter we have highlighted how you can adjust the format of the data within the cells to ensure that Excel interprets it in the correct manner, thus enabling calculations to be undertaken. As well as the number or text format of the cells, Excel also allows for the alteration of the following cell properties:

- alignment of this text;
- font type, size and colour;
- bordering type, weight and colour;
- background colouring.

This can be adjusted manually by selecting 'Format Cells' from the right click option (CRTL+1, CMD+1) on any cell. However, the power of Excel becomes more evident when we combine cell formatting and formulae together to perform formatting based on the values within cells automatically. This is referred to as conditional formatting.

Conditional formatting can be accessed via the 'Styles' group on Windows or the 'Format' group on the Mac. Conditional formatting works by applying rules to the values contained within each cell. By applying conditional formatting to data we can quickly see trends of information and identify ranges of variances in values at a glance. There are some predefined rules already set up in the Conditional formatting, which are very useful.

The 'Conditional Formatting Rules Manager' dialog box allows creation, editing, deleting and viewing of any conditional formatting rules applied to data (Figure 3.17). We can apply these rules individually to specific cells, or to a range of cells. The rules manager allows for multiple rules to be applied to the same cell. When this is done, rules are evaluated in order of their precedence as specified by the order in the list. A rule that is higher up the list will be given a greater precedence over rules further down the list. New rules will be placed at the top of the list by default when they are created, so these will have precedence over already existing ones. We can change the order of these rules by selecting the individual rule and using the 'Move Up' and 'Move Down' arrows.

60

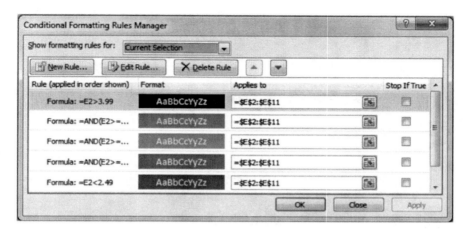

Figure 3.17 The 'Conditional Formatting Rules Manager' dialog box

Table 3.5 Predefined conditional formatting rules

| *Formatting rule* |
| --- |
| Format all cells based on their values |
| Format only cells that contain |
| Format only values that are above or below average |
| Format only unique or duplicate values |
| Use a formula to determine which cells to format |

We may want to use one of the predetermined rules to highlight trends in the data that we have collected. A good analogy is perhaps having traffic light colours to indicate targets for different variables. In order for this to work, we will need to determine the values that form the boundaries for the different colours and use these via the rules of 'Highlight Cells Rules' and 'Greater Than', 'Less Than' or 'Between Values'. This is illustrated in Figure 3.18.

As shown in Table 3.6, we can apply these manually with constant values written into the formula. A better approach to setting up conditional formatting for this traffic light analogy would be to use cell referencing for the boundary values. This way, if we need to change the target values, it is a very quick and easy process.

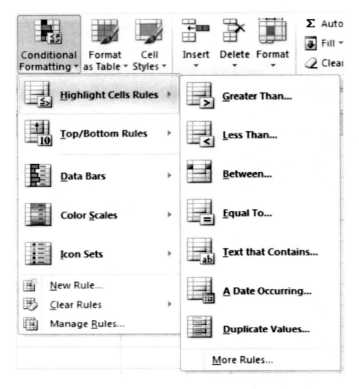

Figure 3.18 Conditional formatting to highlight cells

Table 3.6 Traffic light conditional formatting

| Format | Formatting formula |
|--------|-------------------|
| Green | =P7>3.99 |
| Amber | =AND(P7>=1.99,P7<=3.99) |
| Red | =P7<1.99 |

When one of these predetermined rules is not appropriate for the task we are trying to achieve, we may want to create our own using a formula. By selecting the new rule option, changing the style to 'Classic' and using a formula to determine which cells to format in Excel for Mac we can add our own formula. Alternatively, this can be achieved by selecting new rule, then the rule type of using formula to determine which cells to format in Windows. Here are some examples of formulae that can assist with the formatting of tabulated data. To automatically colour every other row add this formula and adjust the formatting to suit.

=MOD(ROW(),2)=1.

Or to colour every other column

=MOD(COLUMN(),2)=1.

If we are applying multiple formats and conditional formats to cells within our worksheets, we need to think about how these would be handled should conflicts between these rules arise.

**When rules don't conflict**

This is where the rules apply independent formatting options. For example, if one rule formats a cell with a bold font and another rule formats the same cell with a red colour, the cell is formatted with both a bold font and a red colour. Because there is no conflict between the two formats, both rules are applied.

**When rules conflict**

This is where two rules apply the same type of format. For example, one rule sets a cell font colour to red and another rule sets the cell font colour to green. Because the two rules are in conflict, only one can apply. The rule that is applied is the one that is higher in precedence.

**FILTERING AND SORTING**

The data we get from analysis packages is often already sorted chronologically or alphabetically, which in some cases is suitable for further analysis. However, should we want or need to sort or filter the data for other purposes, then Excel makes this possible. It is worth noting that if we are sorting data that contains formulae, the calculation of these data may be affected due to the rearranging of cells.

We can sort data quickly to organise and find the data we want, filter data to display only rows that meet criteria specified, and hide information that we do not want to be displayed. By using conditional formatting that we explored earlier, we can also adjust the format of the data to help visually explore and analyse the data, detect significant issues and identify trends of information (this is further explored in Chapter 4). By combining the sorting, filter and conditional formatting of our data, we can assist in the interpretation by coaching staff and allow them to make more effective decisions based on the data.

## Sorting

To sort our spreadsheet of data, select a single cell within the data range and use **Sort & Filter** from the **Editing Group**. Depending on the type of data in the chosen column, we will get the option of sorting alphabetically A to Z, or Z to A, if numerical data Smallest to Largest or vice versa. The other option that we have is a Custom Sort, where we can also sort the cells via their cell values, cell colour, font colour and cell icon. Note the check box in the top right hand of the Sort dialog box that allows us to indicate whether the data we have selected contain headers or not. If this box is checked it will automatically exclude the first row from the sorting list.

We can also have multiple sorting rules that identify which columns to sort by and when, giving greater control over the organisation of our data. These sorting rules follow a simple hierarchy based on their order. For example, we could sort by more than one cell colour (such as red, then yellow, then green, to indicate different levels of priority) like the traffic light analogy in conditional formatting. Note that if we select more than one cell in a column, Excel will attempt to sort only that range within the column, mismatching the data contained in other columns. Should we try to do this, Excel will indicate a Sort Warning and ask if we want to Expand the selection or Continue with current selection.

We can also sort and filter by using an icon set. Icon sets can be used to annotate and classify data into three to five categories that are separated by threshold values, just like the conditional formatting. Each icon represents a range of values. For example, in the 3 Arrows icon set, the green arrow that points upward represents higher values, the yellow sideways arrow represents middle values, and the red arrow that points downward represents lower values.

64

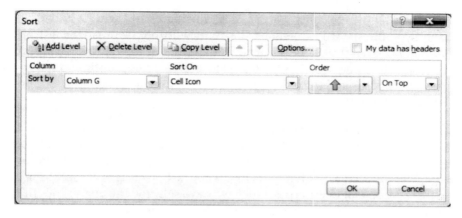

Figure 3.19 Sort via Icon

## Filtering

Using the AutoFilter on our data is a quick and easy way to extract certain smaller datasets from large-scale data. Filtered data displays only the rows of data that meet the specific criteria and hides those that do not. This is useful when we want to display specific data but not remove other data from the dataset entirely.

To use AutoFilter, select any cell on the spreadsheet that contains data and use the **Sort & Filter** button to select **Filter** from the drop-down list. Drop-down menus will then be added to the header row of all the columns that contain data. By clicking on any of the drop-down menus, we will be able to select specific individual variables, or filter types of number or text dependent on the column data type. There are then further filter rules that can be applied (similar to conditional formatting rules) or custom filter rules can be applied.

Unlike sorting, filtering doesn't just reorder the list. It actually hides the rows or columns containing data that do not meet the filter criteria defined.

## CHARTS

Any data that are within our spreadsheets can be graphically represented using charts. Sometimes charts can be more effective at representing the data than tabular formats can be. When using charts within Excel, we have two options: we can embed the chart within the spreadsheet itself, or create the chart on a new sheet. Depending on the context in which we want to show this, we may select a different option. Options surrounding this and the different types of charts will be covered in more detail in Chapter 4.

To create a chart embedded within the same worksheet as the source data, we select the range data we want to chart. We use **Insert** and select one of the chart types from the chart group. We have the option of **Column**, **Line**, **Pie**, **Bar**, **Area**, **Scatter** and **Other Charts**. Selecting one will provide further options for chart types. Once we have selected the chart types that we want, the chart will be displayed within the worksheet.

There are a number of adjustments we can make to the Charts to customise how we want the chart to look. Normally a chart will consist of the graphical representation of the data, data axes, axes titles, legends and chart title. All of these can be individually adjusted to suit. If we want to change the location of the chart, we can right click over the chart and select **Move Chart**, allowing it to either move to a new sheet or be placed within another worksheet as an object.

**Sparklines**

Sparklines are tiny charts within a worksheet cell that provide a visual representation of the data. These can be a nice addition to multiple rows of data to easily show the trends of a series of data values, placed in the same row as the data for more visual impact.

**PROTECTING WORKSHEETS**

When we have spent valuable hours creating a spreadsheet to allow further calculations to be automatically completed from our analysis data exports, we may want to prevent ourselves and other users of the workbook from accidentally or deliberately changing, moving or deleting important formulae, references and charting options. We can do this by protecting certain worksheets or workbook elements, with or without a password.

By default all cells within a spreadsheet are locked when we protect a worksheet. Therefore, when sheets are protected other users cannot insert, modify, delete or adjust the format of data contained in locked cells. When we want other users to be able to use this data sheet, we are going to want them to be able to insert some values in specified cells. To allow this access, before worksheet protection we can unlock the cells so that when the worksheet is locked, these specific cells will allow data entry. To unlock individual cells, select that cell, right click and select **Format Cells** and the **Protection** tab, then uncheck the **Locked** box (this can also be done on a range of cells).

In the same **Protection** tab, we can also specify to hide the formulae within cells. If this **Hidden** box is checked, when the worksheet is protected, the user will not be able to see the formulae contained within. Remember that hiding, protecting and locking elements of the worksheet or the entire workbook will not protect sensitive and confidential data that are contained within. This level of protection merely obscures the data or formulae and prevents users from making changes.

## SUMMARY

Microsoft Excel is a general purpose data analysis package that is widely used by sports performance analysts to process event lists and matrices of results that are produced by commercial video analysis packages. Excel contains a large set of functions for processing numeric and text information. Pre-programmed spreadsheets can be used to analyse sports performance data that can simply be pasted into data areas of worksheets. Pivot tables are particularly useful for cross-tabulating variables, determining counts, means and sums of values. Outputs from spreadsheet processing can be in the form of reports or charts. Conditional formatting allows cells to be automatically coloured to highlight aspects of performance that coaches and players need to pay attention to.

# CHAPTER 4

## DASHBOARDS

### INTRODUCTION

Most readers have probably only come across a dashboard in their cars, and actually this is where the term originated. Drivers can view the important things regarding the function of the car quickly and easily at a glance of the instruments on the dashboard. They tell us all about performance and maintenance needs of the car and allow drivers to ensure that everything is working properly. Now if we move away from the car dashboard metaphor and pull it back to its basic fundamentals we can see that dashboards, in essence, are communicating information. It has been stated that dashboards are a visual display of the most important information parts or parameters needed to achieve key objectives, consolidated and organised onto a single screen to allow all information to be monitored at a glance (Few, 2006; 2013).

Dashboards are used extensively within business intelligence (BI) to display sets of performance indicators (PIs) and key performance indicators (KPIs). The design and function of these dashboards may be focused towards a specific role and display the relevant data. One of the more essential features of such dashboards is the customisable interface and ability to visualise data from multiple different sources. If we look through some samples of dashboards used in the business intelligence environment, we will see that there is a strong preoccupation with gauge-like displays to show data; sometimes with little regard of the data type they display. Oracle and Microsoft are among some of the vendors of BI dashboard software. BI dashboards can also be created through other business applications such as Excel. Figures 4.1 and 4.2 show examples of dashboards from non-sporting domains.

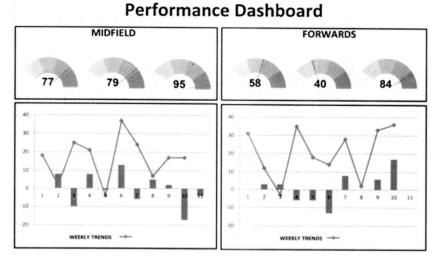

Figure 4.1 Dashboard example

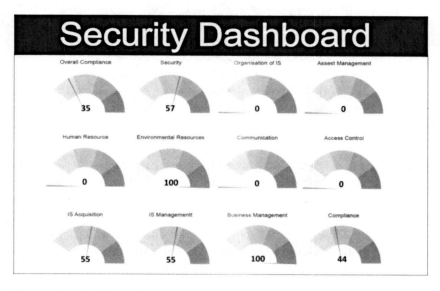

Figure 4.2 Dashboard example

# DASHBOARDS

## What is a dashboard?

Referring back to the definition given by Few (2006; 2013), there are four main facets to understanding the purpose of a dashboard. A dashboard is a visual display, displaying important information based on key objectives, with this information being displayed on a single page in order that it can be viewed and interpreted at a glance.

Visually displaying data, or data visualisation as it has also been termed, has been used for hundreds of years. The most popular forms are the line, bar and pie charts. The information displayed on a dashboard usually includes a combination of text and graphics. The main focus of dashboards is the graphical representation of the data, as if portrayed correctly it can communicate meaning more efficiently than just text.

The data collected via performance analysis is based on performance parameters and objectives, so the translation of the resulting information for dashboard display purposes should be relatively straightforward. What may be more pertinent is deciding which results are the most relevant and worthy of screen real estate. The intended audience may provide direction for the type of information displayed and the manner in which it is presented. However, the important thing to remember is the integration of all this information onto one screen/page. If the viewer has to look between multiple screens/pages to understand the performance data, then this dashboard design has been ineffective. What must also be considered is when the dashboard information is to be used. Readers will see many dashboard examples online that are directly linked to live data. Within the performance analysis arena this may not be desirable, or even possible. However, what we do need to think about is the location of the different sources of information.

Being able to collate data from several different sources isn't necessarily a good thing. Sometimes having too much data can make it more difficult to extract the relevant material for display. What is important to remember is that these dashboards are designed to give an overview of the information. There is a necessity to be all encompassing, providing enough information to highlight trends and identify areas that warrant further investigation via other sources, with the primary purpose of the dashboard being to inform the viewer of what needs to be acted upon.

Creating an effective dashboard is not an easy task. Few people are trained in data visualisation, but yet we all try. Although analysts do not necessarily need to be experts, there are some things that need to be considered first. As screen real estate is limited when displaying information, analysts need to think about the most appropriate mechanism to represent their data to gain optimal impact. Looking at the dashboard examples displayed in Figures 4.1 and 4.2, we can see that they all include a gauge-like design to indicate performance of certain variables. In fact Figure 4.2 only uses this type of data representation. Few (2013) indicated that if the best representation of the data is via gauge-like, traffic signal or thermometer style outputs, then these should be used. However, if there is a better display mechanism, then insisting on similar features found on a car dashboard can be counterproductive.

A combination of several different graphical and tabular types and formats can be used, but what must be foremost in analysts' minds is whether these display outputs communicate the information effectively. Effective communication via graphical and tabular display is not always an intuitive process; what works and is easily understood by one person, does not necessarily translate across to another. The ability to create and design custom dashboards for different purposes is what makes them an attractive prospect for performance analysts. We collect lots of data, producing summary information that different people (coaches, players and other management staff) might want to view. All of these individuals would be viewing this information output for different reasons. So the design and focus could be different for each personnel group.

## Why use dashboards?

It might be important to think about a dashboard as an information display designed to help people maintain situation awareness (SA). This term, originally applied by the military, basically indicates that in order to do a job well we must have constant knowledge of what is going on (Endsley and Jones, 2004). This translates directly to the personnel group with which an analyst would be working. Sometimes we might be able to provide this information live during performances, by using Statistical Output Windows in Sportscode for example (Chapter 5), or at half-time or immediately after the game, by using predesigned Excel spreadsheets (Chapter 3). It is important to remember that situation awareness is based on the facts provided by analysts. Therefore, we must be confident that the information provided is accurate and reliable (Chapter 9).

The reliance of facts regarding a performance is one of the fundamental bases of performance analysis. It has been long known that coaches and game observers struggle to correctly recall and identify important events from a game (Franks and Miller, 1991; Laird and Waters, 2008). We might see events happening, but only a proportion of the details are processed into conscious thought, with yet a further reduction in the amount of detail getting stored as actual memories. So having this important performance information displayed in a clear, precise and usable format is going to be influential to any decision-making process.

The understandings of this information are part of the fundamentals behind the use of dashboards. You have probably heard the saying 'show me the stats', or a derivation of this, several times in many different environments. Certainly in sports, numbers play a central role in the understanding of performance and assist in making important decisions regarding the performance. You would think that numbers are relatively easy to interpret and understand. However, when you are looking at large volumes of information, with several items having the smallest of margins, interpretation can be a difficult.

## Visual perception

Vision is, by far, our most powerful sense. The degree to which a dashboard communicates information effectively and efficiently depends upon the way in which the theories behind visual perception are used. In order to do this, first we must know something about visual perception so that we can manipulate graphics to use these to our advantage.

Visual perception is the way in which our brain and eyes work together in cognitive function to interpret what they see. Vision requires separating foreground from background, recognising different objects and accurately interpreting spatial information. The brain interprets what the eyes are seeing from the light that is focused onto the retina, where it is absorbed by a layer of photoreceptor cells. These cells convert this light into electrochemical signals that are then passed on to the brain. The perception of these signals by the brain is the process of interpreting what we see.

72

We see lots of visual information on a daily basis, but only a fraction of what our eyes see becomes an object of focus. Only a further fraction of these focused objects then become an object of attention, and only a portion of these objects is processed further in conscious thought with a yet smaller portion of stored objects in memory for future use. Without this process of information filtration, what our eyes see would be overwhelming to process (Few, 2013).

Our brains process this information in a similar way to computers. Some of what we see is stored in a temporary memory whilst it is being processed and other things we see are stored for later use. The three fundamental types of memory in the brain are iconic, short-term and long-term. Iconic memory uses a preconscious form of processing known as 'preattentive processing' to filter information to be moved into short-term memory or discarded. Short-term memory is readily accessed but limited in its capacity. Finally, information that is deemed worthwhile for later use is moved into long-term memory for future retrieval.

Visual properties that are processed preattentively, within the working memory, can typically be performed on large-scale data sets in 200 milliseconds or less (Healey, Booth and Enns, 1996). This 'working' or short-term memory has a limited capacity for information storage. This should be taken into consideration when designing dashboards as both individual numbers and line graphs can quickly reach this capacity. Grouping similar items together optimises the use of this limited short-term capacity.

Figure 4.3 highlights a common problem that we would encounter in many team-based sports; separating eleven separate data sets, represented by eleven different coloured lines, cannot be processed into the short-term memory. Instead, the reader would have to constantly refer back to the legend to understand which colour represents which player. To ensure that this process of interpretation is easier, limit the number of data sets used. It would be ideal to group the information about these players, perhaps into playing positions.

Limited sets of visual properties are processed preattentively. It is important to be aware of these to ensure quick and efficient processing of the information on the dashboard. These preattentive attributes are concerned with the form, colour and spacing of visual properties. Some of these attributes are perceptually stronger than others.

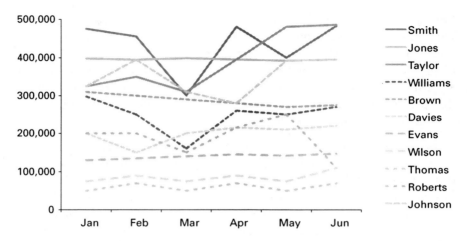

Figure 4.3 Example of graph that exceeds the short-term memory capacity

Consider Figure 4.4. When we perceive colour, we use the saturation and lightness of the colour to differentiate. However, our perception of colours is also interpreted by the influence of the background colour; after all, vision requires the separation of foreground from background.

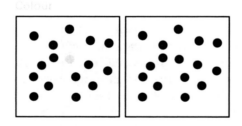

Figure 4.4 Preattentive attributes for colour

In Figure 4.5, all five squares within the rectangle are exactly the same colour as the reference square beneath; all have a colour value of 50% black. In this case, the greyscale gradient fill of the rectangle influences our perception of the colour of the small squares, causing the viewer to perceive them as different shades of grey.

74

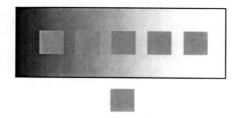

Figure 4.5 Contrast effect on colour perception

Consider the alternative displays shown in Figure 4.6. Line length and line width are extremely useful when interpreting quantitative values indicated inside graphs. Lengths are used to differentiate between values, and can be assisted by scales on the axes. The line width, or weighting as it is sometimes referred to, is useful to highlight different text sections,

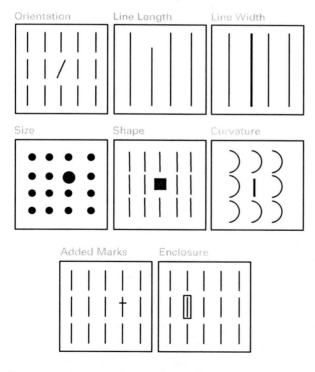

Figure 4.6 Preattentive attributes for form

or provide boundaries around different elements of information, allowing attention to be drawn towards them. It can also be a useful tool to show where some information is grouped together to assist in the noting of relationships between individual information points.

Size of information displayed can be used in two different ways. The size of a graph itself can indicate the relative importance of this information to the viewer. Furthermore, sizes of individual data points within graphs and tables, can assist by showing their relationship with other information. Adding simple markings, shapes or icons into graphs allows easier distinctions to be made and attention to be highlighted.

Position relative to other data points in two dimensional representations is probably one of the easiest preattentive attributes to perceive. This is illustrated in Figure 4.7. This type of representation is used extensively in graphs in order to note where things are in relation to a quantitative scale. This is not easily done when points are placed on a three-dimensional representation, so these should be avoided where possible.

Spatial Position

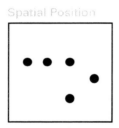

Figure 4.7 Preattentive attribute for spatial position

## DASHBOARD DESIGN

By utilising the knowledge about how visual information is processed by the influence of key preattentive attributes, readers should be able to adequately rise to the challenge of creating an effective dashboard to represent their data. There are two main challenges that dashboard designs must be able to overcome. First, they must be able to show all of the information and make sure that the most important information stands out from the rest. Second, they must be designed and organised in a manner that aids the quick processing, interpretation and understanding of all of the information that is presented.

76

One of the biggest challenges is ensuring that all of the relevant information is being represented, especially as there is limited screen real estate. It is all too easy to litter the dashboard with several graphs and tables that represent information without much thought, just to ensure that the information is there. Remember that what should be presented is based on the performance indicators and performance in relevant areas. This way the dashboard will be more focused, relevant and useful in supporting decisions made (Lewis, 2003).

The dashboard is not supposed to be the only place from where the information can be obtained. This is the first stop for analysts to present performance information. Dashboards can highlight the trends of the performance information, allowing the viewer to identify anything that requires further investigation via other sources. This is the link between the data that have been collected and the corresponding video. If certain areas of performance warrant further investigation, then information filtration processes can be used within the performance analysis packages to retrieve more detailed quantitative information and supporting video sequences.

When displaying quantitative information, it is always pertinent to ensure that we are not wasting visual processing on non-data information. Few (2013) termed this more appropriately for dashboard design as non-data pixels. It refers to the data to pixels ratio when displaying information either in tabular or graphical formats, and relates to any pixels that are not used to display data, excluding the blank background. These non-data pixels should be kept to a reasonable minimum. In Figure 4.8, the three-dimensional element to the bars and the pie charts does not

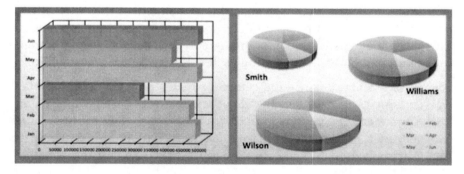

Figure 4.8 Example of excessive percentage of non-data pixels

really add to the information presented; in fact, it actually detracts from the understanding. All the gridlines in the bar chart and the colour gradient can be removed easily without impacting on understanding. Thinking along these principles will help to ensure that dashboards do not become too cluttered with unnecessary visuals that will impact on their efficiency to communicate the information.

## DATA VISUALISATION

Selecting the most appropriate graph or tabular format to represent information via a dashboard is an important task. Analysts need to make sure that it will display the information in the best way and allow for easy and efficient understanding.

### Bar and column graphs

Bar charts and column charts are similar. The main difference is that the bars of a column chart present values in a horizontal direction while the columns of a column chart represent values in a vertical direction. These charts are specifically designed to show multiple measures of information. They are very useful when displaying category-based information, and can show relationships between different measures of information in one clean chart. Charts should not be overcomplicated by adding in numerous gridlines; in fact, some of the most effective charts do not use gridlines at all. When displaying multiple measures on one chart, we should think about the grouping and colours associated with the information. The bar chart works best when displaying information that is either nominal or ordinal in scale, although sometimes they can also be used for interval or ratio-based information categorised into sub-ranges. The individual bars in the bar graph help to delineate between different categories, and assist in separating each value for better interpretation.

Several of the performance indicators for which data are collected may well be associated with elements of performance that have been won and lost. A bar or column chart is ideal for indicating the relationship of these two categories, as they can be placed next to each other for easy comparison. Alternatively, data could always be processed differently (see Chapter 3) so that the information presented portrays the differences between won and lost elements, as shown in the column chart on the right of Figure 4.9.

78

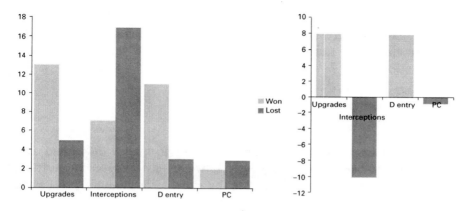

Figure 4.9 Different column charts

When displaying values that represent part of a whole measure, such as percentage of time spent in different pitch zones, a column chart should be used instead of a pie chart. One might think that something that visually represents a whole, like a pie chart, is the most suitable method for this. Figure 4.10 shows the differences between representing the same multiple measures using stacked column charts (sometimes referred to as compound column charts) and pie charts. On the left we can see that the stacked column chart nicely represents information about both teams within one single chart. Two separate pie charts would be needed to

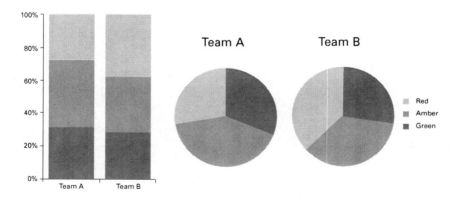

Figure 4.10 Part to whole information representation

represent the same information. The extra space that the radial based graphs, like pie charts and gauges, take up could be better used and multiple pie charts are not necessarily the best method for displaying the information.

**Line graphs**

Line graphs enable us to show changes of performance indicators over time. Like the bar and column charts, they can easily represent multiple measures on one graph. Remember the short-term memory processing limits when selecting the variables to represent; if there are more than five lines on the graph it becomes difficult to distinguish between the lines and recollect which line represents which variable (the right hand line graph in Figure 4.11 is more effective than the line graph on the left). The main difference between the line graph and a column chart is that the variable on the horizontal axis is on a continuous scale. Even though the line graphs in Figure 4.11 show six months, the variables measured on the vertical axis change continuously over time.

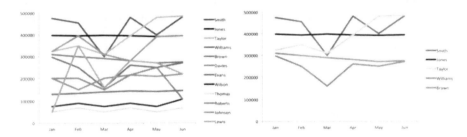

Figure 4.11 Line graphs

**Sparklines**

Developed by Edward Tufte, Sparklines allow for a minimalistic styled line graph to show trends of information over time (Tufte, 2006). Sparklines, often called micro charts, are created within a single cell in

80

Excel and are basically a small line graphic in the form of a graph without the axes. These are often used to add visualisation of information in tabular format without using up too much limited space within the dashboard. Although these Sparklines are quite minimalistic, there are a few formatting options available (Figure 4.12).

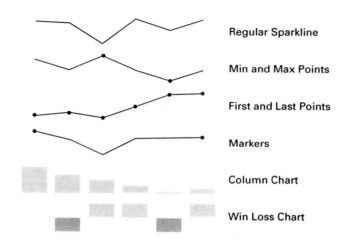

Figure 4.12 Sparklines options

## Bullet graphs

Bullet graphs are, in essence, small horizontal stacked bar charts that have the individual bars overlapped on each other. They were developed by Stephen Few as a more visually appropriate replacement to gauge-like graphics (Few, 2013). These bullet graphs are created using a normal bar chart that is then adjusted to overlap the individual bars. They allow different quantitative ranges to be shown by different colours, with actual and target figures indicated. They have been used alongside Sparklines in tabular based formats.

Sparklines and Bullet graphs are designed to be represented in their simple formats. Just because it may be possible to add lots of extra bells and whistles to them, doesn't mean such additions will be effective.

## Tables

Tables are a simple and effective way to show information in text/value-based formats, but they should be used sparingly. Sets of variables measured using different sub-ranges of numeric values are not suitable for chart representation. The chart would be dominated by variables that use large values. Charts also have problems displaying small differences that can be seen with greater precision within tables. Sometimes it may be beneficial to use tables in conjunction with other graphical based presentation styles to include an extra level of information. As mentioned above, we can also combine the micro charts of Sparklines and Bullet graphs within tables.

## Presentation format

There are a multitude of different output methods that can be employed with the dashboards created. Sometimes analysts will be in direct contact with coaches, players and other personnel on a regular basis. There are other personal who analysts may see more infrequently, but who still have the need to interpret the information. As technology has advanced for the tools that we use to collect the data, so has the technology for the tools available for us to disseminate the resulting information. When creating dashboards, we must always be conscious of how this information is going to be received by these individuals. Analysts may be able to send an electronic copy of a dashboard by email, print it, host it on a website or simply display on a screen (Figure 4.13 shows a smartphone dashboard).

Other considerations are whether we want the information to be static or dynamically linked. By combining the data displayed within the dashboard with a validation list in the spreadsheet (see Chapter 3), we can introduce an element of interactivity to the dashboard with the viewer selecting parts of the information that we wish to adjust, for example we could have individual players statistics.

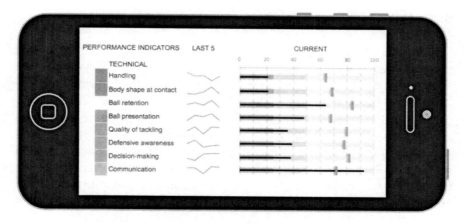

Figure 4.13 Dashboard designed for smartphone display

**Key principles to dashboard design**

■ Make sure to put context to sports performance information. Think about displaying core performance information, such as match teams, half-time and full-time scores.

■ Be purposeful with the selection of information that is displayed. Ask whether the data displayed are relevant performance indicators?

■ Select the most appropriate form of data representation. This needs to quickly and easily communicate the data. Line graphs indicate trends, bar and column charts are good for comparisons.

■ Think about the use of colour and text. Red is easily interpreted as danger or bad, whilst green can be associated with success or good aspects of performance.

■ Group related information together; this aids human memory processing.

■ Don't overcomplicate the visualisation. Simplicity is the ultimate in sophistication. Reduce the volume of non-data pixels and avoid unnecessary text, graphics and gridlines that may cause distractions.

**SUMMARY**

Dashboards are portals of information to the data that analysts have collected using sports performance analysis systems. They should be designed to easily communicate and highlight what the information indicates about the performance. They are designed so that the information can be understood at a glance. When designing dashboards we must always ensure that they are focused for the given audience. They should make use of the chart and table, design and format options available and we should be economical with the screen real estate that they use. Remember, this is the first point of information, so if something is important enough and is highlighted correctly within the dashboard then further investigation into more detailed information and corresponding video can be undertaken.

# CHAPTER 5

## STATISTICAL WINDOWS

### INTRODUCTION

This chapter discusses the Statistical Window of the Sportscode package. Sportscode is used as an exemplar because it is currently the only commercially available sports analysis package that provides a programmable Statistical Window. There are three broad ways of obtaining information from Sportscode once a match has been analysed. First, we can use the Matrix facility, which cross-tabulates events with labels. The Matrix allows us to cross-tabulate events with specifically chosen labels of interest or combinations of labels. These labels are combined using AND, OR and NOT operators. For example, we may wish to see all of the possession events where the outcome was 'Successful' AND the match period was 'Quarter 1' (this has been discussed in Chapter 2). The second way of obtaining information from Sportscode is to export the Event List or the Matrix contents to a general purpose data analysis package such as Microsoft Excel where further analysis of the data can be done. The third way of obtaining information from the Sportscode package is using a Statistical Window. The concept of a Statistical Window is similar to that of a spreadsheet. The Statistical Window contains a table of cells that present text or numeric information. The Statistical Window is programmed to analyse the raw data in the timeline in order to automatically produce information. The Statistical Window can be updated by the user periodically executing the scripts or it can be automatically updated every time there is a change in the timeline. This means that match statistics can be provided live. The information produced can be displayed in the Statistical Window and/or sent to display areas of the

Code Window or an Output Window. Providing match statistics within the Code Window allows analysts to assess areas of performance as they are coding a match. When the statistical information is presented on output windows, it can be viewed by coaches on the bench where areas of the Output Window are sent wirelessly to devices such as iPhones and iPads. This chapter covers the Statistical Window and the script programming language used to program it. A simple example of determining the percentage of possessions that lead to a score is used to illustrate how Statistical Windows access data from the timeline, perform arithmetic operations and send the results to a Code Window. A second example shows how a Statistical Window can be used to determine performance information for individual players in a team game. The third example is a more challenging example that automatically updates the score in a tennis match after each point.

## SCRIPT PROGRAMMING

### Creating a Statistical Window

This section on script programming covers the essential elements of script programming for Sportscode Statistical Windows. However, users are encouraged to read the section on Statistical Windows in the Sportscode manual, which provides a more complete coverage of the available facilities. A Statistical Window is initially created using **File → New → Statistical Window**. A new Statistical Window will appear showing a grid of blank cells. This should immediately be saved and periodically resaved as the Statistical Window is programmed. Unlike Excel, where the default is for rows to be identified by numbers and columns are identified by letters, in a Sportscode Statistical Window both the rows and columns are identified by numbers. Depending on the size of the Statistical Window to be produced, new rows and columns may need to be added. Rows and columns can also be moved or deleted if necessary. The information displayed in a cell can be formatted, made bold, or shown in italics the same way as information in any other package can. Some cells contain scripts that process data while others do not. The cells without scripts are typically areas of the Statistical Window used to display raw values of interest or to display some headings of groups of cells. Where a cell does have a script, the script typically uses the data in the timeline to produce one piece of information that is displayed in that cell. To add or edit a script within a cell, simply press the CTRL key and click on the cell. A menu will appear showing a number of options; select the option 'Edit Script'. This displays a pop up window (an Edit Script window) where the script for the current cell of the Statistical Window is created or edited. The Edit Script window is a text editor allowing scripts to be typed in and edited with cut, copy and paste being allowed the same way as any other text editing (using the Apple Mac computer CMD-X, CMD-C and CMD-V respectively). Once a cell has been programmed with a script, it is distinguished from other cells by having a small triangle marking the top left hand side of the cell. This is important because when we view the Statistical Window, we simply see the information displayed by the cells rather than any function that may have been used to evaluate the information. The triangles tell us where there are scripts that we may need to inspect when developing, debugging or maintaining the system.

## Constants, values and variables

Any data processing or output commands within scripts will use data from the timeline and/or from other cells of the Statistical Window. Let us consider a very simple assignment statement to use raw counts of goals, shots on target and shots off target to compute a higher order variable representing opportunities to score. In Sportscode scripts we use the '$' character as a prefix for all variables. A variable is so called because its value varies; at one time during the match it may hold one value and at another time in the match it may hold another value. We will use $Opportunities as the variable name for scoring opportunities. The following assignment statement uses three literally specified constants to assign the value 11 to $Opportunities. The arithmetic operator '+' is applied to sum the three constants together with the result being assigned to the variable $Opportunities.

$Opportunities = 5 + 4 + 2

This would be of limited use because the assignment command always produces the same answer. It is more likely that we may have other variables to represent the quantities of interest, for example $Goals, $On_target and $Off_target. Each of these variables, like $Opportunities, can hold different values at different times. To assign the sum of their current values to $Opportunities, we would use the following assignment command:

$Opportunities = $Goals + $On_target + $Off_target

The information that we require may be stored in specific cells. For example, cell(6,3) refers to the output (the value currently being displayed) by the cell in the 3rd row and the 6th column. There are also system-provided variables that allow us to specify the current row ($row) and the current column ($column). Imagine that we use a different row for each player with the first five columns of the Statistical Window representing Player Name, Goals, Shots on target, Shots off target and Total scoring opportunities. The cells in the fifth column of the Statistical Window will all be able to use the same script which can be pasted into each cell. The assignment command within each of these cells is as follows:

$Opportunities = cell(2, $row) + cell(3, $row) + cell(4, $row)

This will take the values currently displayed in columns 2 to 4 of the current row and sum them, assigning the result to the variable $Opportunities. It is possible to use a combination of constant values and variables within the same assignment command. For example, the following command determines the percentage of opportunities that resulted in a goal.

$Percentage = 100 * $Goals / $Opportunities

Here, 100 is a constant while $Goals and $Opportunities are variables. Note that '*' is a multiplication operator and '/' is a division operator.


## Assignment commands

We have already seen assignment commands that were used to illustrate the differences between variables and constants. The syntax of an assignment command is:

<Variable> = <Expression>

There must be a variable to the left hand side of the '=' symbol; something that can store the given value. We cannot say 2 = $Goals because the value 2 is always the value 2 and cannot have some other value assigned to it. Variables, on the other hand, are allowed to hold many different values but only one at a time. The expression on the right hand side of the '=' symbol could be a single constant, single variable or some expression in terms of one or more constants and/or variables, the result of which is to be assigned to the variable to the left of the '=' symbol. Consider the following command:

$Goals = $Goals + 1

This does not appear to make sense. How can any number be equal to itself plus 1? The point is that the '=' symbol here does not mean 'is equal to' but means 'becomes'. In other words, the assignment statement evaluates the expression on the right hand side of the '=' symbol and then stores the resulting value in the variable to the left hand side of the '=' symbol. So if $Goals had the value 2 before the assignment command was executed, it will have the value 3 after the assignment command is executed. There is another use of the '=' symbol within conditional statements that will be covered later in the chapter.

Assignment statements are not just used with numerical data but they can also be used with character strings as well. For example, imagine that a player has scored 2 goals from 10 scoring opportunities with these two values being stored in the variables $Goals and $Opportunities respectively. Displaying '20%' in an output window viewed by coaches might not provide sufficient information. The value of 20% could represent 1 goal from 5 opportunities or 40 goals from 200 opportunities. The coaches might also wish to see the number of goals and the number of opportunities. Therefore, we wish to provide an output in the form '2 / 10 = 20%'. This can be done in two steps. First, we determine the percentage of opportunities that resulted in a goal.

$Percentage = 100 * $Goals / $Opportunities

Second, we use an assignment statement where an expression to the right of the '=' symbol constructs a character string in the form '2 / 10 = 20%'. Here we use the variable $String to store the character string.

$String = $Goals + " / " + $Opportunities + " = " + $Percentage + "%"

Note how '+' is used to concatenate character strings together here, while it has been used as an arithmetic operator with numerical variables.

## Accessing data from the timeline

We have seen how to include data within expressions to calculate higher order information such as percentage conversion rates to be displayed for coaches. Ultimately, we need to access raw data from the timeline to include in our calculations. Imagine that we have a code button 'Team A' that represents possessions performed by that team. The following assignment command counts the number of instances in the 'Team A' row of the timeline.

$Possessions = COUNT instances WHERE row = "Team A"

Assuming we have also used labels to show the outcome of different possessions ('Goal', 'On target' and 'Off target'), we can count the number of instances of a given event (code button name) that contain specified value labels. This is done as follows:

$Goals = COUNT "Goal" WHERE row = "Team A"
$On_target = COUNT "On target" WHERE row = "Team A"
$Off_target = COUNT "Off target" WHERE row = "Team A"

If we use a set of value labels to represent different periods in a match ('Quarter 1', 'Quarter 2', 'Quarter 3' and 'Quarter 4'), we could use the following assignment command to determine the number of possessions where goals were scored in a given quarter.

$Q1_Goals = COUNT "Quarter 1" AND "Goal" WHERE row = "Team A"

We can also use the 'NOT' and 'OR' operators in such commands. For example if we wished to count the possessions of Team a that occurred in either the first or second quarter of the match, we would use:

90

$First_half_possessions = COUNT "Quarter 1" OR "Quarter 2" WHERE row = "Team A"

If we were interested in the number of possessions for Team A where a goal was not scored, we could use:

$No_score_possessions = COUNT NOT "Goal" WHERE row = "Team A"

## Timings

As well as counting instances, we can also obtain timing information about the events stored in the timeline. For example, the time at which the last completed possession by Team A ended is given by:

$Last_possession_time_Team_A = END instances WHERE row = "Team A"

The end time of the last completed possession by any team where a goal was scored is calculated as follows:

$Last_goal_time = END "Goal"

The following command will determine the end time of the last instance in the timeline where a goal was recorded for Team A's possessions. Anywhere where the 'END' function is used, it will evaluate to −1 if there are no instances matching the specified criteria.

$Last_goal_time = END "Goal" WHERE row = "Team A"

The function 'START' is similar to 'END' except it determines the start time of the earliest instance in a set of instances.

The LENGTH function allows us to determine the duration (in seconds) of instances. For example if we wished to determine the mean duration of possessions for Team A we would use:

$Total_duration = LENGTH instances WHERE row = "Team A"
$Frequency = COUNT instances WHERE row = "Team A"
$Mean_duration = $Total_duration / $Frequency

Individual instances can be addressed within commands. Instance[2] represents the second instance within a given series of instances while Instance[–2] is the second instance from the end of a series of instances. For example, the length of the most recent possession by Team A would be calculated by the following assignment command:

$Last_duration = LENGTH instance[–1] WHERE row = "Team A"

## Output commands

There are two broad types of output command; the commands that display a resulting value in the current cell of the Statistical Window and the commands that send a value to a display button in a Code Window or Output Window. The 'SHOW' command is used to display the result of a calculation in the current cell. For example, to show the percentage of opportunities by Team A that resulted in a goal, we could do the following:

$Percentage = 100 * $Goals / $Opportunities
SHOW $Percentage

If we have one goal from three scoring opportunities, the resulting percentage might be 33.333333, which we might wish to display using a single decimal place. This can be done with the Round function which rounds up or down for the decimal places not shown or the Floor function which always rounds down. These functions are used expressing the number of decimal places as a second argument with the value of interest being represented by the first argument. For example:

SHOW Round($Percentage, 1)

Or

SHOW Floor($Percentage, 1)

The Round and Floor functions have been used within SHOW commands here, but could have been used within assignment commands prior to the SHOW command.

The second way of providing output is to send a value to a display button in a Code Window or Output Window. Imagine that we have a display button 'Team A PC' in the Code Window that shows the conversion of opportunities by Team A in the form '2 / 10 = 20.0%'. This can be done in two steps. First, we determine the percentage of opportunities that resulted in a goal.

$$\$Percentage = Round(100 * \$Goals / \$Opportunities, 1)$$

Second, we use an assignment statement where an expression to the right of the '=' symbol constructs a character string in the form '2 / 10 = 20%'. Here we use the following commands to construct the character string and SEND to the appropriate button in the code window.

$String = $Goals + " / " + $Opportunities + " = " + $Percentage + "%"
SEND $String to button "Team A PC"

We can also send colours to display buttons in the Code Window or Output Window. The syntax of the command that does this is:

SEND BUTTON COLOR(<red colour>, <green colour>, <blue colour>) TO BUTTON <button name>

The values for red colour, green colour and blue colour can be between 0 and 100 allowing 1,000,000 possible colours. Table 5.1 shows some commonly used colours. So yellow is achieved by using:

SEND BUTTON COLOR(100, 100, 0) TO BUTTON "Team A PC"

Table 5.1 Some display button colours that can be used in SportsCode

| Red colour | Green colour | Blue colour | Resulting colour |
|---|---|---|---|
| 0 | 0 | 0 | Black |
| 0 | 0 | 100 | Blue |
| 0 | 100 | 0 | Green |
| 0 | 100 | 100 | Cyan |
| 100 | 0 | 0 | Red |
| 100 | 0 | 100 | Magenta |
| 100 | 100 | 0 | Yellow |
| 100 | 100 | 100 | White |

## Conditional control – the IF command

There are occasions where we wish to control whether a command is executed or not. For example, consider calculating the percentage of possessions where there was a scoring opportunity. Early in the match there may not be any possessions and so calculating the percentage involves a division by zero error. The 'IF' command can be used to avoid this as follows:

> IF($Opportunities > 0, $Percentage = 100 * $Goals / $Opportunities)

Here, '$Opportunities > 0' is a Boolean expression that evaluates to True or False. If this condition is True then the inner assignment command to calculate $Percentage will be executed. If, on the other hand, this condition is False, then the inner assignment will not be executed.

An alternative form of the 'IF' command involves two inner commands: one to be executed if the condition is True and the other to be executed if the condition is False. The syntax of this form of the 'IF' command is as follows:

> IF(<Condition>, <command to be executed if the condition is True>, <command to be executed if the condition is False>)

'IF' commands can also be nested; this means that the inner commands of an 'IF' command could themselves be 'IF' commands. Let us imagine that we have a display button, 'Team A PC', in the code window that shows the percentage of possessions that lead to a scoring opportunity. If this percentage is greater than 50 per cent we want the display button to be green, if it is less than 25 per cent then we want the display button to be coloured red, otherwise we want the display button to be yellow. This will use the function 'send button color(<red colour>, <green colour>, <blue colour>)'. The following 'IF' command (with an inner 'IF' command sends the appropriate button colour. This is presented here using indentation but the command needs to be typed into a single line in the script editor window.

94

```
IF($Percentage > 50,
        SEND BUTTON COLOR(0,100,0) TO BUTTON "Team A PC",
        IF($Percentage < 25,
                SEND BUTTON COLOR (100,0,0) TO BUTTON
                "Team A PC",
                SEND BUTTON COLOR (100,100,0) TO BUTTON
                "Team A PC"
        )
)
```

## A SIMPLE EXAMPLE

In this section, a simple arbitrary example is used to show how a Statistical Window is used within a system. Figure 5.1 shows the Code Window for this system, which contains two event buttons (Team A and Team B). These two events represent possessions for Team A and Team B respectively. They are exclusively linked because possession alternates between the two teams. The Scored value label is used to record where possessions result in a score for the given team. The final two buttons in the Code Window are used as areas to output statistical information during live coding. Team A PC and Team B PC represent the percentage of possessions that result in a score for Team A and Team B respectively.

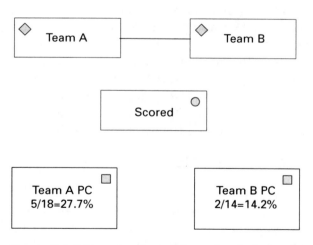

Figure 5.1 The code window for a simple possession analysis system

Figure 5.2 shows the layout of the statistical window used within the system. Column 1 and Row 1 simply contain headings to assist the user reading the results. It is possible to use a single row to determine possessions, possessions that are scored and then output the percentage of possessions that are scored. However, for the purposes of system development and maintenance, it is better that each cell in the statistical window performs a single step in the data processing task. If any errors have been made when programming the scripts in these cells, the intermediate results that are displayed help us determine where the error is so that it can be corrected.

| | Column 1 | Column 2 | Column 3 |
|---|---|---|---|
| 1 | | Team A | Team B |
| 2 | Possessions | 18 | 14 |
| 3 | Scored | 5 | 2 |
| 4 | Percentage | 27.7 | 14.2 |

Figure 5.2 A Statistical Window

Cell(2, 2) determines the number of possessions for Team A. This involves the following two-line script. The first command inspects the timeline and counts the number of instances in the Team A row. The variable $Frequency is a local variable to this cell of the Statistical Window. This means that we can also use the same variable name within Cell(3,2) when determining the number of possessions for Team B. This is because they are two different $Frequency variables, with the scope of each being restricted to the script that they are used within. The second command of the script simply displays the evaluated frequency in the cell.

$Frequency = COUNT instances WHERE row = "Team A"
SHOW $Frequency

Cell(2, 3) determines the number of possessions where Team A has scored. This is evaluated using the following 3 line script. Once again, the variable $Frequency has a restricted scope, which is the current cell and so its value will not be confused with the value of any other $Frequency variable. Cell(3, 3) performs a similar calculation for the number of possessions where Team B score.

```
$Frequency = COUNT "Scored" WHERE row = "Team A"
SHOW $Frequency
```

Cell(2, 4) determines the percentage of possessions where Team A score, displays this in the cell and sends a string in the form '4 / 10 = 40.0%' to the Team A PC display button in the Code Window. The following seven-line script is used to accomplish this.

```
$Frequency = cell($column, $row−1)
$Total = cell($column, $row−2)
IF($Total = 0, Exit)
$Percentage = Round(100 * $Frequency / $Total, 1)
SHOW $Percentage
$String = $Frequency + " / " + $Total + " = " + $Percentage + "%"
SEND $String TO BUTTON "Team A PC"
```

The first two commands simply look up the values being displayed in the two cells above the current cell. The third command is included to prevent the possibility of a division by zero error. It is an IF statement that simply checks if the total number of possessions for Team A is zero and if it is then this execution of the script ceases without the 4th to 7th commands being executed. If Team A have had some possessions of the ball, then commands 4 to 7 are executed. Command 4 determines the percentage. This is done within a round function to ensure the percentage is evaluated to a single decimal place. The 5th command displays the resulting value for $Percentage in the current cell of the Statistical Window. The 6th command builds a character string in the form '4 / 10 = 40.0%' and the 7th command sends this to the Team A PC display button shown in the Code Window (Figure 5.2). We could include an 8th command to control the colour of the Team A PC display button depending on the value of $Percentage. For example, we could use red if the value is less than 30%, green if it is greater than 70% and yellow if it is any other value. This could be done using three separate IF commands or using a single IF command as shown below. Again, note that this command like any other would need to be placed in a single line within the script.

```
IF($Percentage > 70,
        SEND BUTTON COLOR(0,100,0) TO BUTTON "Team A
        PC",
        IF($Percentage < 30,
                SEND BUTTON COLOR(100,0,0) TO BUTTON
                "Team A PC",
                SEND BUTTON COLOR(100,100,0) TO BUTTON
                "Team A PC"
        )
)
```

## INDIVIDUAL PLAYER ANALYSIS

Often we need to produce a Statistical Window to allow statistical results to be compared between players on a team. An example of such a Statistical Window is shown in Figure 5.3.

This Statistical Window shows the frequency of different events performed by different players as well as some percentage success statistics. There are 88 cells arranged in an 8 × 11 array of cells in the Statistical Window. We have two types of script, one that determines the frequency of events performed by a player and one that determines the percentage of events that are performed successfully by the player. This is achieved by placing the player names in the first row of the Statistical Window and the event names in the first column of the Statistical Window. The event names need to be the same as the event names used in the Code Window and hence the same as the names used for rows of the timeline. Similarly, the player names need to be the same as the value labels used for players in the timeline.

If each of the 66 frequency cells refers to the location of the event type and player name relatively rather than absolutely then the same script can be used in each cell. An additional advantage of this is that if a player name changes for a subsequent match, the analyst only has to change the player name in the first row of the Statistical Window.

Consider the shaded cells in column 7 of the 6th and 7th rows. The following script is used to determine the frequency of tackles performed by Ed in the first of these two cells. This is because cell($column, 1) is the first cell and the current column (Ed) and cell(1, $row) is the 1st cell

98

in the current row (Tackle). This script can now be copied into rows 2, 4, 8 and 9 within the same column (column 7) to determine the frequency of passes, shots, interceptions and dribbles performed by Ed.

```
$Frequency = COUNT cell($column, 1) WHERE row = cell(1,
$row)
SHOW $Frequency
```

For those cells where a percentage success value needs to be calculated, the following script is used. Any events of the given type where the player of interest and 'Successful' are included as labels will be counted by the second command of this script. This script is keyed into the second shaded cell (row 7 and column 7) in Figure 5.3 and the script copied into cell(7,3) and cell(7,5) so that we also have the percentage success for passes and shots.

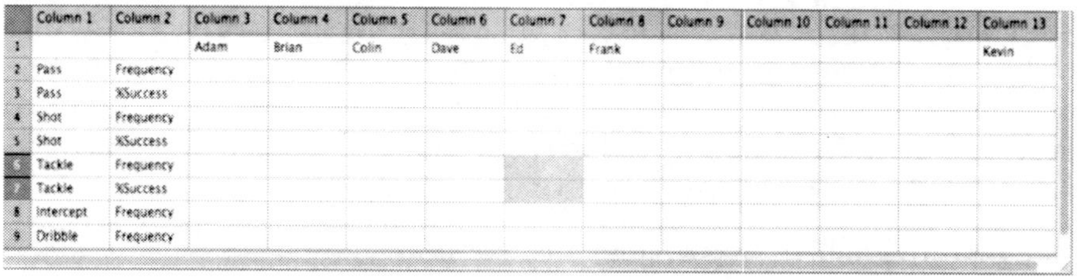

| | Column 1 | Column 2 | Column 3 | Column 4 | Column 5 | Column 6 | Column 7 | Column 8 | Column 9 | Column 10 | Column 11 | Column 12 | Column 13 |
|---|---|---|---|---|---|---|---|---|---|---|---|---|---|
| 1 | | | Adam | Brian | Colin | Dave | Ed | Frank | | | | | Kevin |
| 2 | Pass | Frequency | | | | | | | | | | | |
| 3 | Pass | %Success | | | | | | | | | | | |
| 4 | Shot | Frequency | | | | | | | | | | | |
| 5 | Shot | %Success | | | | | | | | | | | |
| 6 | Tackle | Frequency | | | | | | | | | | | |
| 7 | Tackle | %Success | | | | | | | | | | | |
| 8 | Intercept | Frequency | | | | | | | | | | | |
| 9 | Dribble | Frequency | | | | | | | | | | | |

Figure 5.3 Layout of Statistical Window for individual player statistics

```
$Total = COUNT cell($column, 1) WHERE row = cell(1, $row)
$Frequency = COUNT cell($column, 1) AND "Successful"
WHERE row = cell(1, $row)
IF($Total = 0, Exit)
$Percentage = Round(100 * $Frequency / $Total, 1)
SHOW $Percentage
```

To copy an entire column (or row) including the scripts to another column hold down the ALT and CMD keys and then drag the column (or row) header to the new location that it is copied to. This saves a lot of time when creating large Statistical Windows where the same scripts are used in multiple columns (or rows). In this example, our column 7 will have been completed first and then copied in its entirety into columns 3 to 6 and 8 to 13.

## AUTOMATIC UPDATE OF SCORE IN TENNIS

### System Requirements

Consider a tennis match between players A and B where A is serving at 1–1 in sets, 5–6 in games and 15–40 in points. Imagine that Player B wins the point; what is the score now? If you understand tennis, you will know that this means that Player B not only wins the point but also wins the game and wins the set 7–5. This also means that the next point will be the first point of a new game where player B is serving instead of player A. Because the score in tennis can be determined from the score at the beginning of the point and knowledge of who wins the point, it should be possible for a computerised system to automatically update the score, which will save the user needing to do this during data entry. This brings us to a fundamental principle of using Statistical Windows, which is that anything that can be determined automatically should be determined automatically. This not only reduces the data entry load on system operators but also prevents user some errors during data entry.

The requirements of this system are as follows:

■ To allow tagging of points with the user identifying the start and end of points as well as the winning player.
■ The system updates the score and serving player automatically. To make this system a simpler example than it might otherwise be, tiebreakers are not played.
■ The Code Window must include a display area showing the server and the current score in sets, games and points.
■ The scores of completed sets (in games) are to be shown in display buttons within the Code Window.

A more complicated version of the system can be attempted by readers to include tie-breakers. If readers are attempting this, a hint is to: (a) use a cell to represent whether the match is the best of three or five sets; and (b) use another cell to represent whether a tiebreaker is played in the final set or not.

# 100

## System design

Figure 5.4 shows the Code Window for the tennis system. There are event buttons to record the start (Serve) and end (End Point) of points. The End Point event is used to represent the inter-point breaks that start as soon as a point ends. For each point we need to enter a label representing the point winner (Player A or Player B) before entering End Point. The cells with square symbols to the top right are all display buttons used to display the serving player and the current score. The current score is shown comprising of serving player, set score, game score and points score. At the bottom of the Code Window we have an area where previous set scores are retained. This is a different format of showing the score which repeats game and point information shown earlier in the code window.

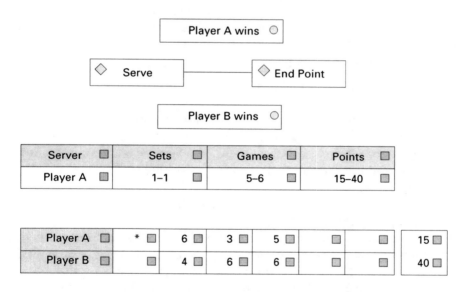

Figure 5.4 The code window for the tennis system

Figure 5.5 shows the structure of the Statistical Window. The shaded cells (with the exception of row 1 and column 1) contain scripts that evaluate different variables for the score and display these. Rows 8 and 9 are

| | Column 1 | Column 2 | Column 3 | Column 4 | Column 5 | Column 6 | Column 7 |
|---|---|---|---|---|---|---|---|
| 1 | | Before Point | Before Point | After Point | After Point | | |
| 2 | | Server | Player A | Server | Player A | | |
| 3 | | Server | Receiver | Server | Receiver | Carry | |
| 4 | Sets | 0 | 0 | 0 | 0 | 0 | |
| 5 | Games | 0 | 0 | 0 | 0 | 0 | |
| 6 | Points | 0 | 0 | 0 | 0 | | |
| 7 | | Server | Set 1 | Set 2 | Set 3 | Set 4 | Set 5 |
| 8 | Player A | * | 0 | | | | |
| 9 | Player B | | 0 | | | | |

Figure 5.5 Structure of the Statistical Window for the tennis system

used to show the score in previous sets as well as the current server (denoted by an '*'). The first 6 rows show the score in sets, games and points noting the serving player. Within these 6 rows, columns 2 and 3 show the score at the beginning of the point while columns 4 and 5 show the score at the end of the point.

There are 6 steps in the algorithm which are outlined as follows:

1 When the user presses the Serve button to start a new point, the Statistical Window copies the score at end of previous point into the score at the start of the current point. The Serve event deactivates any inter-point break event that had been active before the current point commenced.

2 The user indicates whether Player A or Player B won the point using the appropriate label.

3 Having entered the point winner, the user presses End Point to complete the Serve (point) event. This starts off a series of tasks that the Statistical Window performs automatically in steps 4 and 5.

4 The Statistical Window determines the score at the end of the point using detail of the player who won the point and the score at the beginning of the point. The Serving player for the next point is also determined.

5 The Statistical Window sends the updated score to the appropriate display buttons in the Code Window.

6 Now we are back to Stage 1 waiting for the user to press the Serve (point) button to start the next point.

102

The order in which cells are evaluated for the score after the point is points score first, then game score and then set score. This is because we may win a game as a result of winning point and we may win a set as a result of winning a game. We cannot assume that a point score of 0–0 (Love All) means a game has just been won. This is because the first point in the match is a special case. So the system uses cell(6,5) and cell(6,4) to 'carry' a game or a set in the same way that we use carry when doing long addition. The difference here is that cell(6,5) could be +1 if the server has just won the game, −1 if the server has just lost the game and 0 if the current game is continuing in the next point. Cell(6,4) does the same task when winning (or losing) a game means that the server wins (or loses) the set.

**The scripts**

The Statistical Window uses 0, 1, 2, 3, ... to represent points within games but these are output as Love, 15, 30, 40, ... in the relevant display buttons of the Code Window. The first cells that we will consider in the Statistical Window are the cells in columns 2 and 3 that store the score before the point is played. As soon as a new point starts (step 1 of our 6 step process), the score displayed at the end of the previous point is copied into the cells displaying the current point. The following script is used for each of the seven cells to be updated; the server, the sets for the serving and receiving players, the games for the serving and receiving players and the points for the serving and receiving players. The value to be displayed is initially assigned as the currently displayed value. The second command changes the value by copying the value in the cell that is two columns to the right of the current cell. This is only done if a point is being played; that is the 'Serve' button is active because a point is being recorded into the timeline. BUTTON "Serve" STATE is evaluated to True if the button is pressed down (active) and False if it is up. The $value is then displayed in the current cell.

```
$value = cell($column, $row)
IF(BUTTON "Serve" STATE, $value = cell($column+2, $row))
SHOW $value
```

In the same way that the score at the beginning of the point is only updated when the 'Serve' button in the Code Window is active, the score at the end of the point is only updated when the 'End Point' button in the Code Window is active. The cells evaluating the score at the end of the point inspect the timeline to see who won the point and the score at the beginning of the point in order to evaluate a component of the score after the point. The following script is for cell(6,4) which evaluates the points score for the server. Here we need to know about the server's and receiver's points score before the point ($sp_pre amd $rp_pre) in order to determine the server's points score after the point ($sp_post). The first command sets up a variable to represent the player who served the point. The second command determines whether 'Player A wins' is a label in the last instance recorded in the timeline (instance[−1] is the last recorded instance in the timeline). If this is the case then Player A won the point otherwise Player B won the point. The 3rd command simply evaluates a Boolean expression asking whether the serving player is the same as the player who won the point. The truth of this comparison is stored in the variable $serverwins. Commands 4 and 5 set up variables for the points won by the serving and receiving player within the game before the current point started. The 6th command is a bit complicated and applies if the serving player won the point. If the serving player had more than two points before the current point started and was leading by at least one point then winning the current point means that the serving player has also won the game. Therefore, the point score for the serving player after the game would be 0 otherwise it would be one greater than it was at the beginning of the point. The 7th command does something similar if the receiving player won the point. The 8th command of this script ensures that the computed value for $sp_post is only displayed in the cell, if we are in an inter-point break. Cell(5,6) contains a similar script that determines the receiver's points score after the point ($rp_post).

```
$server = cell(3,2)
IF(count label "Player A wins" IN instance[−1], $winner="Player
A", $winner="Player B")
$serverwins = ($server = $winner)
$sp_pre = cell(2,6)
$rp_pre = cell(3,6)
IF($serverwins,
        IF(($sp_pre>2)AND(($sp_pre − $rp_pre)>0),
                $sp_post=0,
                $sp_post = $sp_pre+1
```

```
            )
    )
    IF($serverwins=0,
            IF(($rp_pre>2)AND(($rp_pre − $sp_pre)>0),
                    $sp_post=0,
                    $sp_post = $sp_pre
            )
    )
    IF(BUTTON "End Point" STATE, SHOW $sp_post)
```

If the points score (cell(4,6) and cell(5,6)) has been set to 0–0, then cell(6,5) needs to 'carry the 1 or −1' so that we know whether to update the game score or not. The following script is stored in cell(6,5). The first four commands place the server's and receiver's points scores before and after the point into local variables. The 5th command determines whether the server has won or lost the game or whether the game continues in the next point. If the points score is recorded as 0–0 both before and after the point it is because we are at the beginning of the match and no point has been played yet. If, however, the score after the point is 0–0 but the score before the point was not 0–0, then someone has won the game. This is determined by whether the server or receiver was winning the game before the point started. The local variable $gamewinner represents the carry value which could be 0 if we are still in the same game, −1 if the server has lost the game or +1 if the server has won the game.

```
    $sp_pre = cell(2,6)
    $rp_pre = cell(3,6)
    $sp_post = cell(4,6)
    $rp_post = cell(5,6)
    IF(($sp_post=0)AND($rp_post=0),
            IF(($sp_pre=0)AND($rp_pre=0),
                    $gamewinner=0,
                    IF($sp_pre>$rp_pre,
                            $gamewinner=1,
                            $gamewinner=−1
                    )
            ),
            $gamewinner=0
    )
    IF(BUTTON "End point" STATE, SHOW $gamewinner)
```

Once we know whether a game has been won or lost by the server, we can update the server for the next point in cell(5,2). This is done using the following script. The value of $gamewinner is inspected in the first command; this will be −1, 0 or +1 depending on whether the server has lost the game, the game continues or the server won the game respectively. The second command stores the name of the serving player at the beginning of the point in the variable $server_pre. If the game continues in the next point then $server_post is simply assigned the value of $server_pre. If, on the other hand, the game has just finished, then it does not matter which player won the game because the player to serve in the next point will be different to the player who served in the last point of the current game. As before, changes to post point score variables are only made if we are in an inter-point break. This is dealt with by the fourth command in the script.

```
$gamewinner =cell(6,5)
$server_pre = cell(3,2)
IF($gamewinner = 0,
        $server_post=$server_pre,
        IF($server_pre = "Player A",
                $server_post = "Player B",
                $server_post = "Player A"
        )
)
IF(BUTTON "End point" STATE, SHOW $server_post)
```

The 'carry' information about whether a game has just been won or lost by the serving player is also used by the script in cell(4,5) which determines the serving player's game score at the end of the current point. In order to determine the game score for the serving player after the point we need to inspect the game score for the serving ($sg_pre) and receiving ($rg_pre) players at the beginning of the point. The script computes the game score for the serving ($sg_post) and receiving ($rg_post) players at the end of the point. This is done in commands 6 to 9 of the script. Here, if a player had won a game as a result of winning the point, had won more than four games before the point had started and had a lead of at least one game before the point started, then the player has just won the set. If this happens, the game score for both players needs to be set to 0–0. If winning the point does not mean that one of the players has just won the set, but has won the game, we simply add 1 to the game score for that player. This is because the serving player will be switched to the other player if the game has just ended. The commands 10 to 12 are only executed if the game has just ended; that is if $gamewinner is not equal to 0. Note the '!=' symbol is the 'is not equal to' operator. These three commands swap the game scores for the two players if a game has just ended because we always specify the new server's score first. The script for cell(5,5) which determines the receiver's games after the end of the point is similar.

```
$gamewinner = cell(6,5)
$sg_pre = cell(2,5)
$rg_pre = cell(3,5)
$sg_post = $sg_pre
$rg_post = $rg_pre
IF($gamewinner=1,
        IF(($sg_pre>4)AND(($sg_pre-$rg_pre)>0),
                $sg_post=0,
                $sg_post = $sg_pre+1
        )
)
IF($gamewinner=1,
        IF(($sg_pre>4)AND(($sg_pre-$rg_pre)>0),
                $rg_post=0,
                $rg_post = $rg_pre
        )
)
IF($gamewinner=-1,
        IF(($rg_pre>4)AND(($rg_pre-$sg_pre)>0),
                $sg_post=0,
                $sg_post = $sg_pre
        )
)
IF($gamewinner=-1,
        IF(($rg_pre>4)AND(($rg_pre-$sg_pre)>0),
                $rg_post=0,
                $rg_post = $rg_pre+1
        )
)
IF($gamewinner != 0, $temp = $rg_post)
IF($gamewinner != 0, $rg_post = $sg_post)
```

```
IF($gamewinner != 0, $sg_post = $temp)
IF(BUTTON "End point" STATE, SHOW $sg_post)
```

By winning a point, we might win a game and might also win a set. A value of −1 or +1 is displayed in cell(6,4) to indicate if a set has just been completed; −1 would mean the serving player just lost the set while +1 would mean the serving player has just won the set. The following script sets up the 'carry' value in cell(6,4). The first four commands copy the game score before and after the point into local variables which are then used within the 5th command. The 5th command checks if the game score after the previous point is 0–0. If the game score after the point is 0–0 then comparing the game scores before the point ($sg_pre and $rg_pre) will tell us whether someone has won the set. If a set has just been completed then $setwinner is determined (−1 for the receiver winning the set and +1 for the server winning the set). This value is then displayed in cell(6−4)

```
$sg_pre = cell(2,5)
$rg_pre = cell(3,5)
$sg_post = cell(4,5)
$rg_post = cell(5,5)
IF(($sg_post=0)AND($rg_post=0),
        IF( ($sg_pre=0)and($rg_pre=0),
                $setwinner=0,
                IF($sg_pre>$rg_pre,
                        $setwinner = 1,
                        $setwinner = −1
                )
        ),
        $setwinner = 0
)
IF(BUTTON "End point" STATE, SHOW $setwinner)
```

The sets scoreline after the match can now be determined. The set score for the serving player is determined in cell(4,4). This uses the following script. We need to know if someone has just won a set ($setwinner) in order to update the set score. We also use the fact that someone has just won a game to swap the server's and receiver's set scores in commands 9 to 11, because the other player will be serving in the next game. Commands 3 and 4 retrieve the set score before the point while

# 108

commands 5 and 6 initially set the set score at the end of the point to be the same as it was before the point in case there are no changes. Commands 7 and 8 update the set score while commands 9 to 11 swap the two players' set scores after the point because the other player will be serving the next point as it will be the first point of a new set.

```
$setwinner = cell(6,4)
$gamewinner = cell(6,5)
$ss_pre = cell(2,4)
$rs_pre = cell(3,4)
$ss_post = $ss_pre
$rs_post = $rs_pre
IF($setwinner = 1, $ss_post = $ss_pre+1, $ss_post = $ss_pre)
IF($setwinner = −1, $rs_post = $rs_pre+1, $rs_post = $rs_pre)
IF($gamewinner != 0, $temp = $ss_post)
IF($gamewinner != 0, $ss_post = $rs_post)
IF($gamewinner != 0, $rs_post = $temp)
IF(BUTTON "End point" STATE, SHOW $ss_post)
```

The longest script in the statistical window is in cell(5,4) which not only evaluates the receiver's set score at the end of the point but is able to send values to display buttons in the Code Window now that the whole score after the point has been determined. This script contains 41 commands and so it is discussed in sections. The first 11 commands are similar to evaluating the set score for the serving player. It is actually only the last command that differs in that it shows the receiving player's set score rather than the serving player's.

```
$setwinner = cell(6,4)
$gamewinner = cell(6,5)
$ss_pre = cell(2,4)
$rs_pre = cell(3,4)
$ss_post = $ss_pre
$rs_post = $rs_pre
IF($setwinner = 1, $ss_post = $ss_pre+1, $ss_post = $ss_pre)
IF($setwinner = −1, $rs_post = $rs_pre+1, $rs_post = $rs_pre)
IF($gamewinner != 0, $temp = $ss_post)
IF($gamewinner != 0, $ss_post = $rs_post)
IF($gamewinner != 0, $rs_post = $temp)
IF(BUTTON "End point" STATE, SHOW $rs_post)
```

The next part of the script sends the score with respect to the player serving in the next point to the grid of eight cells in the middle of Figure 5.4 (these are the cells that show the score Player A serving at 1–1 in sets, 5–6 in games and 15–40 in points). The names of the display buttons are shown in italics in Figure 5.4. The first two commands set up local string variables to represent the serving and receiving player at the beginning of the next point. The serving player's name is then sent to the button 'ServerName'. The 4th command constructs a string to represent the set score including the number of sets won by player separated by a hyphen. This is sent to the 'SScore' display button in the code window.

```
$server = cell(5,2)
IF($server = "Player A", $receiver = "Player B", $receiver = "Player
A")
SEND $server to BUTTON "ServerName"
$setscore = $ss_post + "−" + $rs_post
SEND $setscore TO BUTTON "SScore"
```

The next four commands perform a similar task for the game score, accessing it from the two cells where it is stored in the Statistical Window, creating a string to represent the game's score and sending this to the 'GScore' display button in the code window.

```
$sg_post = cell(4,5)
$rg_post = cell(5,5)
$gamescore = $sg_post + "−" + $rg_post
SEND $gamescore TO BUTTON "GScore"
```

Displaying the points score in the 'PScore' button of the Code Window is a little more challenging because we wish to use 'Love', '15', '30', '40', … instead of 0, 1, 2, 3, … when presenting the score. Therefore, we use nested IF commands to transform the server's numerical point score ($sp_post) into a value to be displayed ($sp_disp). This is also done for the receiving player.

```
$sp_post = cell(4,6)
$rp_post = cell(5,6)
IF($sp_post = 0,
        $sp_disp = "Love",
        IF($sp_post = 1,
```

```
              $sp_disp = "15",
              IF($sp_post = 2,
                      $sp_disp = "30",
                      $sp_disp = "40"
              )
      )
)
IF($rp_post = 0,
      $rp_disp = "Love",
      IF($rp_post = 1,
              $rp_disp = "15",
              IF($rp_post = 2,
                      $rp_disp = "30",
                      $rp_disp = "40"
              )
      )
)
```

These string values can be used if the point score is before the first deuce score in the game. Where the game has already reached the first deuce, the score will be one of 'Deuce', 'Adv Player A' or 'Adv Player B'. The level of nesting of IF commands means that this is better presented here using indentation, but it does have to be keyed into the script editor window as a single line of text.

```
IF($sp_post+$rp_post < 6,
      $pointscore = $sp_disp + "–" + $rp_disp,
      IF($sp_post>$rp_post,
              $pointscore = "Adv " + $server,
              IF($sp_post<$rp_post,
                      $pointscore = "Adv " + $receiver,
                      $pointscore = "Deuce"
              )
      )
)
SEND $pointscore TO BUTTON "PScore"
```

Having sent the points score to the 'PScore' display button, we also need to send the two players' individual point scores to the 'AP' and 'BP' display buttons (see Figure 5.4). If the score is 'Deuce' we display '40' in each of these display buttons. If the score is advantage to one player then we use an 'A' for the player's score and '40' for the opponent's score. If the score has not yet reached the first deuce in the game then we can simply send $sp_post and $rp_post to the 'AP' and 'BP' display buttons.

```
IF($sp_post+$rp_post > 5,
        IF($sp_post>$rp_post,
                $sp_disp = "A",
                $sp_disp = "40"
        )
)
IF($sp_post+$rp_post > 5,
        IF($rp_post>$sp_post,
                $rp_disp = "A",
                $rp_disp = "40"
        )
)
IF($server = "Player A",
        SEND $sp_disp TO BUTTON "AP",
        SEND $rp_disp TO BUTTON "AP"
)
IF($server = "Player B",
        SEND $sp_disp TO BUTTON "BP",
        SEND $rp_disp TO BUTTON "BP"
)
```

The final task of the script in cell(5,4) is to check if the current set has been completed and if a game score of 0–0 needs to be placed in the next set of the code window. If we have just completed the first set, then we need to send 0 to the display buttons 'A2' and 'B2' to set the score at the start of the second set to 0–0. If a later set has just been completed we need to send 0 to the display buttons 'A3' and 'B3' or 'A4' and 'B4' or 'A5' and 'B5'. A set has been completed if the 'carry' cell(6,4) is –1 or +1. The value is compared to 0 and the result stored in the local variable $setover. If the score in sets is 1–1 then the next set is the third set as set up in the second command below.

```
$setover = ($setwinner != 0)
$nextset = $ss_post + $rs_post + 1
IF(($setover != 0)AND($nextset = 2), SEND 0 TO BUTTON "A2")
```

```
IF(($setover != 0)AND($nextset = 2), SEND 0 TO BUTTON "B2")
IF(($setover != 0)AND($nextset = 3), SEND 0 TO BUTTON "A3")
IF(($setover != 0)AND($nextset = 3), SEND 0 TO BUTTON "B3")
IF(($setover != 0)AND($nextset = 4), SEND 0 TO BUTTON "A4")
IF(($setover != 0)AND($nextset = 4), SEND 0 TO BUTTON "B4")
IF(($setover != 0)AND($nextset = 5), SEND 0 TO BUTTON "A5")
IF(($setover != 0)AND($nextset = 5), SEND 0 TO BUTTON "B5")
```

Rows 8 and 9 of the Statistical Window are used to place the score of completed sets in the display buttons 'AS', 'BS', 'A1', 'B2' through to 'A5' and 'B5'. We will show the scripts for two of these cells. Firstly, cell(2,8) is used to show an '*' character if Player A is serving, otherwise it is left blank. The script for this cell is as follows. The script for cell(2,9) performs a similar process for Player B.

```
$server = cell(5,2)
IF($server = "Player A", $marker = "*",$marker = " ")
SHOW $marker
SEND $marker TO BUTTON "AS"
```

Finally, we will consider cell(5,8) which places Player A's number of games in the current set in the display button 'A3'. This is done when each game within the 3rd set ends. The 10 cells from cell(2,8) to cell(7,9) all have similar scripts to this. Take a close look at the 11th command below '$serverwon = ($ss_post>$rp_pre) OR ($sg_post>$rg_pre)'; it does not look right does it? A player has won the game if the player has more games after the point than before the point or, if the new game score is 0–0 at the start of a new set, the player has more sets after the point than before. Command 12 appears to be comparing the player with the other player! Remember, if a game has just ended then the player who is serving now was receiving in the previous point. So command 12 is actually comparing the same player's score before and after the point that has just been played. Command 14 is another strange one. We are taking the game score prior to the point and adding one to the game winner's number of games before the point. This is because if someone has just won the set 6–4, we never actually see 6–4 in the current score which has already been changed to 0–0 in the next set. We are not corrupting the game score before the point because the variables $sg_pre and $rg_pre only have scope within cell(5,8). These are then used to determine what value to display in the display button 'A3'. The value displayed is $sg_pre if

Player A was serving and $rg_pre if Player A was receiving. Command 16 sets up a Boolean variable $can_display which used in the final two commands of the script to control whether or not the set score is displayed in this cell and display button 'A3'. The set score is only displayed if we are indeed in the 3rd set, a game has just ended and the match is in an inter-point break.

```
$server = cell(5,2)
$gamewinner = cell(6,5)
$gameover = ($gamewinner !=0)
$ss_pre = cell(2,4)
$rs_pre = cell(3,4)
$ss_post = cell(4,4)
$rs_post = cell(5,4)
$sg_pre = cell(2,5)
$rg_pre = cell(3,5)
$sg_post = cell(4,5)
$rg_post = cell(4,5)
$serverwon = ($sg_post>$rg_pre) OR ($ss_post>$rp_pre)
$set = $ss_pre + $rs_pre
IF($serverwon,
        $sg_pre = $sg_pre + 1,
        $rg_pre = $rg_pre + 1
)
IF($server = "Player A",
        $display_games = $sg_pre,
        $display_games = $rg_pre
)
$can_display = $gameover AND ($set = 3) AND (BUTTON "End
point" STATE)
IF($can_display, SHOW $display_games)
IF($can_display, SEND $display_games TO BUTTON "A3")
```

This was a challenging Statistical Window to create. Adding tiebreakers and ensuring the Statistical Window works correctly for best of three sets and five sets matches and whether or not a tiebreaker is used in the final set present further challenges that some readers may like to take up. The author has developed a further version of this Statistical Window to address these issues but feels that the version presented here is more suitable to illustrate Statistical Windows.

# 114

## OTHER COMMANDS

The commands covered in this chapter process data from the timeline. There are other useful commands that perform operations on areas of the Statistical Window itself. We have seen how to change the colour of display buttons in the Code Window to highlight some aspect of performance. CELL_COLOR allows us to change the colour of a cell in the Statistical Window. The PUSH BUTTON command allows the Statistical Window to automatically push code buttons or value label buttons DOWN or UP. For example, we could have a series of 18 value labels representing the game scores from 'Love-Love' to 'Deuce', 'Advantage Server' and 'Advantage Receiver'. The statistical window could push these buttons at the beginning of each point so that each point in the timeline had a value label for the game score at the beginning of the point. This would save the user having to enter these labels and would facilitate analysis of performance in particular scorelines.

## SUMMARY

The Statistical Window in Sportscode can be programmed to analyse the timeline and automatically calculate information, saving system operator time. The information produced in the Statistical Window can be sent to display buttons in the Code Window or in separate Output Windows. The Statistical Window can also activate and deactivate buttons in the Code Window. Developers should use Statistical Windows to ensure that anything that can be calculated automatically is calculated automatically. This will make the system operator's task easier and reduce data entry errors. However, programming a Statistical Window is time consuming and the effort needs to be justified. The decision about using a Statistical Window depends on how often the system is going to be used. This chapter has covered some of the facilities provided in Statistical Windows. Readers are encouraged to read the Sportscode user manual and help files provided by Sportscode and to try these in their own systems. This will develop further practical skill and problem solving ability.

# CHAPTER 6

## PLAYER TRACKING DATA

### INTRODUCTION

There are different types of player tracking technology, which have been discussed in recent reviews (Carling *et al.*, 2008; Carling and Bloomfield, 2013; Leser and Roemer, 2014). Some systems are fully automated while others require some human verification activity of data. The accuracy of systems varies and some may be considered useful for sports such as orienteering and sailing but not for team games played on a restricted playing surface. Some systems can be used indoors while other systems can only be used outdoors. This is particularly the case with GPS systems. The accuracy of systems is increasing as technology develops over time. Therefore, the current chapter is neither based on a particular technology nor rules out any technology. The idea is to describe the analysis of player tracking data that have been captured by a system that is assumed to be accurate and reliable.

The main commercial systems, such as Prozone3 (Prozone Sports Ltd, Leeds, UK), have been used to provide various types of information about tactical and physical aspects of movement. The movements of players can be animated on a bird's-eye view of the pitch in one part of the system interface while another part of the screen shows corresponding match video. The visual information from player tracking systems allows collective movement of players to be analysed qualitatively (Dijk, 2011). The systems can also show the locations of accelerations, decelerations and high speed runs. Quantitative information about distance covered in different speed zones can be produced with the threshold values for running, high-speed running and sprinting being tailored for individual player abilities. Player tracking data have been analysed to automatically recognise occurrences of different types of cutting movement (Robinson *et al.*, 2011). There has also been some research done using player tracking data to quantify tactical aspects of play. Some of these have looked at movement of team centroids (Lames *et al.*, 2009; Lemmink and Frencken, 2011; Duarte *et al.*, 2011) while others have analysed spatial distributions of players (Fonseca *et al.*, 2013; Robles *et al.*, 2011). These studies were largely exploratory and a much greater volume of data would be needed to establish whether such variables distinguish between possession plays of differing outcomes. Areas of soccer performance with the potential for automatic analysis using player tracking data can be identified by reviewing books on soccer coaching and tactics. Some of these text books have been available for decades but the tactical events described have not been introduced into systems analysing player tracking data. There are attacking aspects such as penetration, which can be recognised from changes in player locations over short periods of time (Worthington, 1980; Hargreaves and Bate, 2010). Defending aspects related to the balance of the defence have been described by Olsen (1981) and Tenga (2010). Concentration of the defence (Worthington, 1980) refers to the concentration of players in areas that need to be defended rather than the psychological skill of concentration. Other aspects of defence in soccer coaching literature that have the potential for automated analysis are compactness of the defence (Daniel, 2003) and the use of zonal and man-to-man marking (Prestigiacomo, 2003). Player tracking data can be analysed with respect to movement made over time, meaning that concepts such as delaying have the potential to be analysed using the data (Worthington, 1980). Depth and width of teams is relevant to attacking and defending (Daniel, 2003). Teams are trying to create space when attacking (Bangsbo and Peitersen, 2004) and, when defending, they are trying to restrict the space that opposing teams have to play in (Bangsbo and Peitersen, 2002). Gréhaigne *et al.* (1997) used Amisco data (Amisco, Nice, France) to identify areas covered by players moving at different speeds. The idea is that there is a trade-off between how far a player can move and how much they can change direction. When the player is moving fast they can move further but have limited scope for changing direction. When moving slowly there is greater ability to change direction but the distance that can be reached in the next 1 second is limited by the initial speed the player is moving at.

The automated analysis of player tracking data has been limited. At the 8th International Symposium of Computer Science in Sport, Lames and

Siegle (2011) and O'Donoghue (2011) called for more ambitious use of player tracking data to provide information on tactical aspects of play that are relevant to coaching. Many of the tactical movements described in soccer coaching literature can potentially be recognised through automated analysis of player tracking data. O'Donoghue (2011) reported on an algorithm developed to measure variables related to the balance of the defence according to Olsen's (1981) principles. This is illustrated in Chapter 7 when discussing the use of Matlab. For an algorithm to be developed to automatically analyse any aspect of play, there must be: (a) an understanding of aspect of play; (b) precise definitions of location and movement patterns that characterise the aspect of play; and (c) a mathematical representation of the aspect of play. The overall approach used in the current chapter involves the following five stages:

- Selection of an aspect of play to be analysed automatically
- Operationalising the aspect of play
- Specifying the process (WHAT the algorithm will do)
- Designing and implementing the algorithm (HOW the algorithm works)
- Validation of the process

The current chapter follows these stages using the example of challenging in soccer. Initially, we need to select the tactical aspect of play to be analysed automatically. This involves considering the coaching context, referring to stakeholders and reading soccer coaching books that describe the aspect in order to justify that it is relevant and important. The approach at this stage is vague as it is first necessary to consider the tactical area of interest broadly, determining if it can be analysed automatically using player tracking data and identifying the types of output required and how these may assist in coaching.

The tactical area of interest can then be operationalised by defining the conditions necessary for recognising it. In the case of challenging, what we really need to know is when a dribble counts as a challenge and when it does not. It is necessary to specify the criteria that must hold for a dribble to count as a challenge. These criteria then need to be expressed rigorously in terms of the data structures that are available for analysis. The specification of the process also needs to consider the format of the outputs produced. The algorithm does not merely identify challenges (or whatever other tactical event may be of interest) but it also produces information required about these events. There may be measurable characteristics of tactical events that are required at an individual event level, player performance level or relating to the team performance as a whole. The specification of the system should be completed before commencing any programming. The specification provides a sound understanding of what is required of the algorithm and helps communication between developers and users allowing clarification of requirements where necessary.

Once the specification is agreed, the algorithm can be implemented. The current chapter recommends a data oriented approach rather than a fine-grain object oriented approach. Thus we are developing an algorithm and any necessary intermediate data structures to fulfil the task. Once the algorithm has been developed and tested for correctness with respect to the specification, it needs to be validated. The difference between verification and validation is that validation is concerned with whether the process actually identifies the tactical events of interest whereas verification only considers this with respect to our operational definition of the tactical event. Validation typically involves users identifying events of interest from video observation of matches and comparing these with the events identified by the algorithm that used the player tracking data. There will always be some loopholes in definitions that mean some of the events that are really performed in matches do not satisfy the criteria set for the algorithm to recognise them. Similarly there may also be occasions where an event is recognised by the algorithm, correctly applying the operational definition being used, but which practitioners would not consider as qualifying as a counting event.

## PLAYER TRACKING DATA

Player tracking data typically includes the X and Y locations of each player at frequent time intervals during a match (for example Prozone3 records these data at 10 Hz). This is a valuable source of accurate movement data that can be used for many different types of scientific investigation as well as providing useful information for practical coaching. However, one of the major obstacles to producing meaningful information from the player tracking data is that these data alone do not provide information on which team or player is in possession of the ball or whether the match is in live game time or stoppage time at any moment. However, additional data relating to possessions and on-the-ball events can be provided from different sources and augmented to the player tracking data. Indeed, Prozone provides separate systems for the analysis of player movement and for the analysis of on-the-ball events. The current chapter proposes an approach of analysing player movements that also makes use of on-the-ball event data. This has been done before for analysis of spatial characteristics of play (Lames *et al.*, 2013). The current chapter proposes using such an approach in the automatic identification of specific event types that have been discussed in soccer coaching literature. Figure 6.1 shows the relationship between the data processing algorithm and existing systems. The match event data and the player movement data will have already been produced by existing systems and so the data processing algorithm must use these data in the form in which they are provided. This may involve some data transformation if a third party company has produced such an algorithm to use with data from many different player tracking technologies.

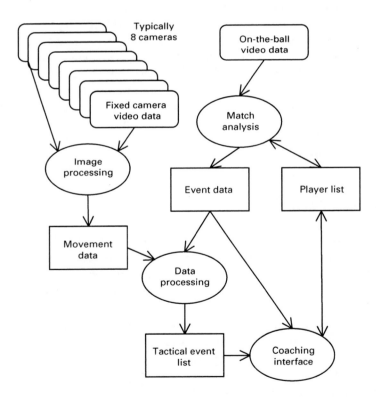

Figure 6.1 Components of a combined player tacking/match analysis system

120

The output of the algorithm needs to be a list of timed recognised tactical events that can be provided on the system interface the same way as any other event type. In Prozone, the acceleration events, deceleration events and on-the-ball match events are all clickable events on a bird's-eye view image of the pitch. This might require the new events to be added to the existing match event list. However, it is more likely that it would be kept separate but in a consistent form that the system interface can use if this event type is selected. This is because the match event list is an important data file in its own right without the augmented tactical events provided by the types of algorithm discussed in the current chapter. The Player List allows the system to be used with multiple matches by naming the given 14 players of each team (11 starting players and up to 3 substitutes) who take part in a match. The player codes used in other data structures link to these player names that can then be provided on interfaces during data entry or analysis. There are other global variables used to help analyse individual match data. These include a variable representing the direction of play of each team in the first half as well as variables for the dimensions of the pitch which may differ between matches.

## CHALLENGING IN SOCCER

The event type that has been chosen for use as an example in this chapter is 'challenging' in soccer. Bangsbo and Peitersen (2004: 31–3) described challenging as dribbling the ball towards an opponent, forcing the opponent to defend the space they are in and this creates space for the dribbling player's teammates. In Figure 6.2, player A has the ball and dribbles towards the opponent C creating space for player B to move into.

Challenging can also involve a change of tempo (Bangsbo and Peitersen, 2004: 33) with the dribbling player increasing running speed when close to the opponent to dribble past the opponent or luring the opponent to follow the dribbling player. This may involve a change of direction, as shown in Figure 6.3, and the ball may be passed when the player gets close to the opponent or shortly after if the opponent has been lured away from space where the player wishes to pass the ball. Dribbling the ball towards an opponent does risk losing possession of the ball and the risk increases the later the player leaves it before passing the ball. Bangsbo and Peitersen (2004: 32) listed four aims of challenging an opponent:

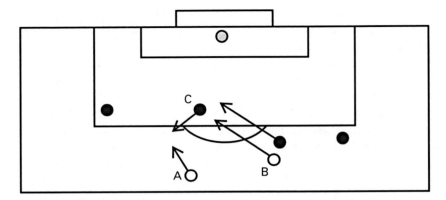

Figure 6.2 Player A challenges opponent C to make space for teammate B

1   to dribble the ball past the opponent and create an attacking situation where the team have superior numbers to the opposing team;
2   to utilise free space;
3   to create free space for teammates;
4   to demonstrate courage by dribbling the ball directly towards an opponent.

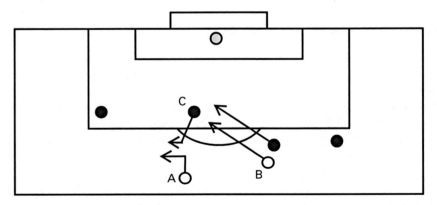

Figure 6.3 A challenge involving a change of direction

One or more of the dribbling player's teammates should move in a way that makes them available to receive the pass in open space. This may involve moving towards the area where the challenge is being made or away from the area. There are some vague terms in Bangsbo and Peitersen's (2004) description of challenging. For example, it is appropriate for the player with the ball to make a challenge if the opposing defence is badly organised and the nearest opposing defender is moving forward. The term 'badly organised' is something that may be analysed subjectively and so won't be used in the current example.

## OPERATIONALISING EVENTS

The current example is limited to challenges that take opponents away from the player to be passed to. The analysis is concerned with three main players (the dribbling player, the teammate to be passed to and the challenged opponent). The other defending players are examined during the process of identifying the challenged opponent and determining the amount of space a player has before and after the dribble. The first step in developing the algorithm is to establish criteria for a dribble to count as a challenge. These are initially specified in vague terms as we gradually move from the coaching problem domain to the program implementation domain. The following seven criteria for a challenge to be identified are listed:

1   there is a dribble event followed by a pass;
2   the dribbling player is in the opponent's half;
3   the dribbling player moves forward;
4   the closest opponent is goal-side of the dribbling player;
5   the closest opponent at end of dribble is closer to the dribbling player than at the start of the dribble;
6   the teammate receiving the ball after the dribble has more space than at the start of the dribble;
7   the closest opponent was closer to the space eventually passed to by the dribbling player at the start of the dribble than at the end of the dribble.

There are some measurable properties of challenges that vary between challenges that may be required as outputs or may be used for exploratory research to compare the types of challenge made by successful and less successful teams. These include:

1   the space difference for the dribbling player before and after the dribble;
2   the space difference for receiving player before and after the dribble;
3   the length of the dribble;
4   the speed of dribbling.

Some aspects of challenges not dealt with by the algorithm but that may be considered during qualitative analysis of video sequences of identified challenges are the directness of the challenge to the opponent as well as the pace change and direction change of the dribbling player as the distance to the challenged player closed.


## SPECIFICATION

### Data structures

The match event data in this example are stored as a two-dimensional array of records called Match. The array is indexed by half of the match (1 or 2) and the event number (1, 2, 3, 4 ...) within the half. The event records within each half are stored in chronological order and contain seven fields:

- the time of the event in seconds from the beginning of the given match period (measured to the nearest 0.1s);
- the event type (e.g. pass, shot, tackle, dribble);
- the team performing the event;
- player code (1–14) for the player performing the event;
- player2 code (1–14) for the second player involved in the event (recorded for some event types);
- the X coordinate of the pitch location of the event;
- the Y coordinate of the pitch location of the event.

Therefore, the type of event performed in the 17th event of the first half is given by Match[1,17]. Event while the location of the event is given by Match[1,17].X and Match[1,17].Y.

# 124

The player codes are used to locate players in a file of player names that are relevant for the current match. This is a file of two columns, one for each team, and 14 rows, one for each player within each team who participated in the match. If fewer than three substitutes were used then the appropriate cells are left blank to represent this. There are global variables of Pitch_Length and Pitch_Width, which are initialised to represent the dimensions of the pitch the current match is being played on, for example 114m and 80m respectively.

The location of events is represented by X and Y coordinates. X represents the back to forward location on the pitch with values ranging from –Pitch_Length / 2 to Pitch_Length / 2 (–57m to +57m for example) and 0m being the halfway line. Y represents the width of the location and ranges from –Pitch_Width / 2 to Pitch_Width / 2 (–40m to +40m for example with –40 representing the left side line the team playing towards the goal line at +57m for example). Thus, the coordinates (0,0) represent the centre of the pitch.

The player tracking data are stored in a separate data structure, Loc, to the match event data. This is a four-dimensional array indexed by half (1 or 2), time (tenth of a second within the half), team (home or away) and player (1 to 14). Each record contains 3 values:

- playing – which is a Boolean (true or false) variable indicating whether the player is on the pitch or not at the given time;
- the X coordinate of the pitch location of the player;
- the Y coordinate of the pitch location of the player.

Therefore, the location of player 9 of the home team at 5 mins and 30s of the second half would be addressed as Loc[2, 3300, Home, 9].X and Loc[2, 3300, Home, 9].Y. The 3300 is the number of tenths of seconds that have elapsed within the second half after 5 mins and 30s.

A tactical event list is produced by the algorithm allowing the identified challenges to be used by output and analysis facilities provided to the users. This part of the process will not be covered in detail within the current chapter as it is a straightforward building of a list of start and end times with additional information representing the movement during the challenge.

## Direction of play

If we wish the algorithm to work for teams playing in either pitch direction, we either need to double the amount of program code by repeating the same basic program code within the 'THEN' and 'ELSE' parts of an IF statement or we need some way of representing direction. We can have a variable, DIR, which is either −1 or +1, depending on the direction the home team is playing in during the first half. We can simply use this as a multiplying factor within the code to allow the code to be used for play in both directions. By multiplying by this 'Direction' variable, we effectively rotate the pitch by 180° in one case so that all events can be considered as if played in the same direction.

## ALGORITHMIC DESIGN

Rather than using a specific programming language, this chapter uses pseudocode (structured English) to express the algorithm used as an example. The algorithm evaluates whether an event numbered, Event_No, within a match period, Half, is a challenge or not. At the highest level, the algorithm is expressed as a function that uses lower-level functions for the criteria used to recognise a challenge. The lower-level functions are Boolean functions used with local variables representing the players potentially involved in a challenge being evaluated. There are 7 of these lower-level Boolean functions, one for each of the criteria for a challenge identified earlier in the chapter. Two of the criteria can be checked using the same Boolean function but called with different parameters. Specifically, the Closer_After function can be used to determine if the dribbling player is closer to the challenged opponent afterwards as well as being used to determine whether the teammate receiving the pass is closer or not to the challenged opponent after the dribble than before. There is also a procedure to determine the challenged player. The difference between a function and a procedure is that a function is evaluated to a value, preferably without changing any existing variables while a procedure can change or initialise variables. In this case, the procedure Determine_Challenged_Opponent determines the opponent it is believed has been challenged by the dribbling player if the other criteria hold. One of the seven functions, Opponent_Goalside, is called from within this procedure rather than the top level Is_Challenged function. The Is_Challenged function does use some local

126

variables, which are provided as arguments to the lower level functions. These are:

- Dribbling_Player
- Receiving_Player
- Challenged_Opponent
- Att_Team
- Def_Team

If all of the criteria for a dribble being a challenge hold then the function is evaluated to True, allowing details of the recognised challenge to be added to the Tactical Event List used in analysis facilities provided to users.

```
FUNCTION Is_Challenge(Half, Event_No)
BEGIN
    IF Dribble_then_Pass(Half, Event_No) THEN
        {* Determine Team and Player performing dribble *}
        Dribbling_Player = Match[Half, Event_No].Player
        Att_Team = Match[Half, Event_No].Player
        Def_Team = Other(Att_Team)
        Receiving_Player = Match[Half, Event_No +
        1].Player2
        IF    In_Opponent_Half(Half, Event_No, Att_Team,
              Dribbling_Player)
              AND
              Dribbling_Forward(Half, Event_No, Att_Team,
              Dribbling_Player)
        THEN
              Determine_Challenged_Opponent(Half,
              Event_No, Challenged_Opp)
              IF    (Challenged_Opp > 0) AND
                    Closer_After(Half, Event_No, Att_Team,
                    Dribble_Player,
                        Def_Team, Challenged_Opp) AND
                    More_Space_After(Half, Event_No,
                    Receiving_Player) AND
                    NOT Closer_After(Half, Event_No,
                    Att_Team,
                        Receiving_Player, Def_Team,
```

```
                           Challenged_Opp)
                 THEN
                        RETURN TRUE {* This is a challenge *}
                 ELSE
                        RETURN FALSE
                 ENDIF
          ELSE
                 RETURN FALSE
          ENDIF
      ELSE
          RETURN FALSE
      ENDIF
   END FUNCTION
```

The function Other is used to determine the other team. This is used in various lower level functions for the criteria of challenging as well as in the overall Is_Challenge function.

```
   FUNCTION Other(Team)
   BEGIN
          IF Team = Home THEN
                 RETURN Away
          ELSE
                 RETURN Home
          ENDIF
   END FUNCTION
```

The first criteria is assessed by simply looking at the match event data and checking if the two events starting at a given event in a given half are a dribble and then a pass performed by the same team. The function needs to check that there is an event after the one numbered Event_No within the half to avoid a run time error for trying to read beyond the end of the file.

```
   FUNCTION Dribble_then_Pass(Half, Event_No)
   BEGIN
          {* Need to make sure there is an event after to avoid run
          time error *}
          IF Event_No is the last event in the half THEN
                 RETURN FALSE
```

```
            ELSE
                    IF      Match[Half, Event_No].Event = Dribble AND
                            Match[Half, Event_No+1].Event = Pass AND
                            Match[Half, Event_No].Team = Match[Half,
                            Event_No+1].Team
                    THEN
                            RETURN TRUE
                    ELSE
                            RETURN FALSE
                    ENDIF
            ENDIF
      END FUNCTION
```

The function In_Opponent_Half is the first to use the DIR variable, which indicates the direction of play of the home team in the first half. If the home team are playing 'from left to right' (from negative values of X to positive values of X) in the first half, then DIR is +1 otherwise it is −1. What we initially need to do is determine the direction of play for the given team in the given half. This is done by a lower level function TEAM_DIR which is invoked by In_Opponent_Half among other functions.

```
      FUNCTION TEAM_DIR(Team, Half)
      BEGIN
            IF Team = Home THEN
                    IF Half = 1 THEN
                            RETURN DIR
                    ELSE
                            RETURN −DIR
                    ENDIF
            ELSE
                    IF Half = 1 THEN
                            RETURN −DIR
                    ELSE
                            RETURN DIR
                    ENDIF
            ENDIF
      END FUNCTION
```

We could assess whether the dribble and pass events are within the opponent's half by using the match event data or the player location data. The two sets of data should be reasonably consistent although there may be a slight difference between the location of an event recorded by the operator of a match analysis system and the location of the player concerned as recorded by a player tracking system. In this function, the match event data are used. We multiply the result of TEAM_DIR function by the X location of the dribble and pass events being performed and if the result in each case is positive then the team is in the opponent's half.

```
FUNCTION In_Opponent_Half(Half, Event_No, Team, Player)
BEGIN
        IF    (TEAM_DIR(Team, Half) * Match[Half, Event_No].X
              > 0) AND
              (TEAM_DIR(Team, Half) * Match[Half,
              Event_No+1].X > 0)
        THEN
              RETURN TRUE
        ELSE
              RETURN FALSE
        ENDIF
END FUNCTION
```

Similarly, the Dribbling_Forward function could use match event data for the location of the start of the dribble and the pass that followed it. Such data are satisfactory for very broad decisions such as in which half of the pitch an event occurs, but the detail required to make decisions about movement during dribbles would benefit from more accurate player tracking data. Therefore, the Dribbling_Forward function uses event times to access the relevant locations of players that have been recorded.

We need to consider what we mean by a dribble going forwards. Do we mean getting closer to the goal line, irrespective of whether travelling towards the goal or the corner flag, or do we mean getting closer to the centre of the goal. In the Dribbling_Forward function we assume the latter. The function uses a general distance function based on Pythagoras' Theory.

# 130

```
FUNCTION Distance(X1, Y1, X2, Y2)
BEGIN
        RETURN SQRT( (X1-X2)^2 + (Y1-Y2)^2 )
END FUNCTION

FUNCTION Dribbling_Forward(Half, Event_No, Team, Player)
BEGIN
        {* Convert event times in secs to times in tenths of secs to
        address Loc array *}
        Start_Time = Match[Half, Event_No].Time * 10
        End_Time = Match[Half, Event_No+1].Time * 10
        {* determine dribbling player location before and after
        dribble *}
        X_before = Loc[Half, Start_Time, Team, Player].X
        Y_before = Loc[Half, Start_Time, Team, Player].Y
        X_after = Loc[Half, End_Time, Team, Player].X
        Y_after = Loc[Half, End_Time, Team, Player].Y
        {* the location of the centre of the opponent's goal *}
        X_Goal = TEAM_DIR(Team, Half) * Pitch_Length / 2
        Y_Goal = 0
        {* Determine if distance to goal is reducing *}
        Dist_to_goal_at_start = Distance (X_before, Y_before,
        X_Goal, Y_Goal)
        Dist_to_goal_at_end = Distance (X_after, Y_after, X_Goal,
        Y_Goal)
        RETURN Dist_to_goal_at_end < Dist_to_goal_at_start
END FUNCTION
```

There are many different approaches for determining the player who was challenged. The dribbling player should be taking the ball towards them and then passing the ball to a teammate. We could identify the opponent closest to the dribbling player on average during the dribble. Alternatively we could assume that it is the player the dribbling player is closest to at the end of the dribble. It is this latter approach that is used in the Determine_Challenged_Opponent procedure. The half and event number of the dribble event are input arguments to this procedure. Challenged_ Opp is an output argument whose value is initialised by the procedure. The times used in the match event list are in seconds and so they need to be multiplied by ten to determine the number of tenths of seconds which is used to index the Loc array containing the player tracking data.

```
PROCEDURE Determine_Challenged_Opponent (INPUT Half,
                                          Event_No,
                                          OUTPUT
                                          Challenged_Opp)
BEGIN
      {* Determine teams and players involved *}
      Att_Team = Match[Half, Event_No].Team
      Def_Team = Other(Att_Team)
      Dribbling_Player = Match[Half, Event_No].Player
      {* Convert event times in secs to times in tenths of secs to
      address Loc array *}
      End_Time = Match[Half, Event_No+1].Time * 10
      {* determine dribbling player location before and after
      dribble *}
      X_after = Loc[Half, End_Time, Att_Team,
      Dribbling_Player].X
      Y_after = Loc[Half, End_Time, Att_Team,
      Dribbling_Player].Y
      {* Search for closest goal-side opponent at the end of the
      dribble *}
      Closest_Distance = Infinity
      Closest_Opponent = 0 {* if this remains 0 then there is no
      goalside opponent *}
      FOR opp = 1 TO 14 DO
            {* is the opponent on the field *}
            IF Loc[Half, End_Time, Def_Team, opp].Playing
            THEN
                  X_opp = Loc[Half, End_Time, Def_Team,
                  opp].X
                  Y_opp = Loc[Half, End_Time, Def_Team,
                  opp].Y
                  {* Is the opponent goal side *}
                  IF Opponent_Goalside(Half, End_Time,
                  Att_Team, Dribbling_Player, Def_Team, opp)
                  THEN
                        Dist_to_opp = Distance(X_after, Y_after,
                        X_opp, Y_opp)
                        IF Dist_to_opp < Closest_Distance
                        THEN
                              Closest_Opponent = opp
```

```
                    Closest_Distance = Dist_to_opp
              ENDIF
        ENDIF
      END
  ENDFOR
  Challenged_Opp = Closest_Opponent {* passed out as an
  output parameter *}
END PROCEDURE
```

The Determine_Challenged_Opponent function uses the Opponent_Goalside function as it searches for the closest goalside opponent to the dribbling player at the end of the dribble. The Opponent_Goalside function simply determines the distance between a player and the centre of the goal that the team in possession is attacking. This distance is calculated for the dribbling player and the current opposing player being considered. If the opposing defender is closer to the goal they are defending then they are considered to be goalside of the dribbling player. This definition of goalside is open to criticism because a defender could be closer to their goal than the dribbling player but be on the left of the penalty area while the dribbling player is on the right. The function could be elaborated to check that the defending player is within a triangle formed by the dribbling player and the goal posts. However, this can be criticised because a defender might be to one side of this imaginary triangle as they try to prevent the dribbling player from shooting with their dominant foot. In the current algorithm, the use of the Opponent_Goalside function for each defending player along with the distance they are from the dribbling player is expected to overcome the problem of a defender being 'goal side' but on the other side of the penalty area. Figure 6.4 illustrates this. Player A is dribbling the ball and there are three opponents who are goalside of him (opponents C, D and E). Opponents D and E are closer to the goal than opponent C, but opponent C is the closest goalside opponent to player A. Therefore opponent C is counted as the challenged player.

The FOR loop is used to look at each on-field opponent changing the closest goalside opponent as successive opposing players are looked at finding closer opponents than the closest found so far. However, further calls of the Opponent_Goalside function will be made for closer defenders to the dribbling player. This may seem like a very trivial and detailed consideration, but readers developing tactical analysis algorithms are

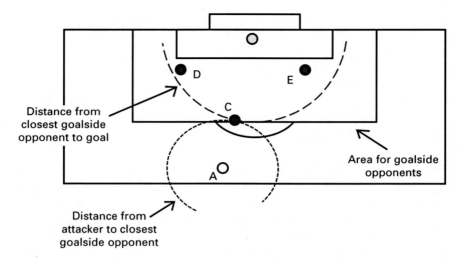

Distance from closest goalside opponent to goal

Area for goalside opponents

Distance from attacker to closest goalside opponent

**Figure 6.4** Alternative goalside opponents

encouraged to consider the algorithms they are developing in this way. They should always be asking 'is there a pattern of players that would trick my algorithm into recognising an event by mistake?' Developers can simply draw patterns of players on paper and deliberately try to achieve such a pattern that would be counted as a given tactical event by the algorithm but which the developers and coaches would not count. When they do produce such patterns they need to consider whether the criteria for the algorithm need to change or whether the case is too rare to be addressed by the criteria.

```
FUNCTION Opponent_Goalside(Half, Time, Att_Team, Player,
Def_Team, Opp)
BEGIN
        {* the location of the centre of the opponent's goal and the
        two players *}
        X_Goal = TEAM_DIR(Att_Team, Half) * Pitch_length / 2
        Y_Goal = 0
        X_Player = Loc[Half, Time, Att_Team, Player].X
        Y_Player = Loc[Half, Time, Att_Team, Player].Y
        X_Opp = Loc[Half, Time, Def_Team, Opp].X
        Y_Opp = Loc[Half, Time, Def_Team, Opp].Y
```

# 134

{* Determine if opponent is goalside *}
Dist_player_to_goal = Distance (X_Player, Y_Player, X_Goal, Y_Goal)
Dist_opp_to_goal = Distance (X_Opp, Y_Opp, X_Goal, Y_Goal)
RETURN Dist_opp_to_goal < Dist_player_to_goal
END FUNCTION

The Closer_After function is used to determine if the distance between two players is closer at the end of the dribble than before. The function is actually called twice within the root level Is_Challenge function; once to determine if the dribbling player is closer to the challenged defender afterwards and once to check that the receiving player is NOT closer to the challenged defender after the dribble than before. The function simply uses the Distance function to apply Pythagoras' Theory to determine the distance between the two players both before and after the dribble and then simply compares these distances.

```
FUNCTION Closer_After(Half, Event_No, Team1, Player1,
Team2, Player2)
BEGIN
        {*      Are the two players closer when the next event is
                performed than they are when the current event is
                performed – first we need to check that there is a
                next event *}
    IF Event_No is the last event in the half THEN
                RETURN FALSE
    ELSE
                {* Determine the times of the event and following
                event *}
                Start_Time = Match[Half, Event_No].Time * 10
                End_Time = Match[Half, Event_No+1].Time * 10
                {* Determine co-ordinates *}
                X1_before = Loc[Half, Start_Time, Team1, Player1].X
                Y1_before = Loc[Half, Start_Time, Team1, Player1].Y
                X2_before = Loc[Half, Start_Time, Team2, Player2].X
                Y2_before = Loc[Half, Start_Time, Team2, Player2].Y
                X1_after = Loc[Half, End_Time, Team1, Player1].X
                Y1_after = Loc[Half, End_Time, Team1, Player1].Y
                X2_after = Loc[Half, End_Time, Team2, Player2].X
```

Y2_after = Loc[Half, End_Time, Team2, Player2].Y
{* Determine distances between players and compare them *}
Dist_before = Distance(X1_before, Y1_before, X2_before, Y2_before)
Dist_after = Distance(X1_after, Y1_after, X2_after, Y2_after)
RETURN Dist_after < Dist_before
        ENDIF
    END FUNCTION


## VALIDATION

The tactical events identified by an automated algorithm need to be validated against expert human classification of such events. The automated algorithm is deterministic and will produce the same set of results no matter how many times it is applied to the same player tracking data. Human classification of tactical events, on the other hand, involves subjective processes and we, therefore, need some evidence that human classification of tactical events is reliable. At least two expert human observers are needed to classify tactical events during video observation. Their results can then be compared with those of the automated algorithm used to identify tactical events using player tracking data. Where there are two observers, we will have three data sets to compare as illustrated in Table 6.1. The data in Table 6.1 are fictitious data that are used to illustrate how an algorithm can be validated. Table 6.1(a) shows reliability results for the human classification of tactical events. The match may contain 20 dribbles according to the match event data and so video sequences of these 20 dribbles are viewed independently by the two human observers. They classify each dribble as being a challenge or not. Observer 1 and Observer 2 classify 8 and 9 dribbles respectively as being challenges but they only agree that a dribble is a challenge for 7 of these. The kappa value can be computed and interpreted, in this case, as a good strength of agreement ($0.60 \leq \kappa < 0.80$) (Altman, 1991: 404). There will be understandable reasons why some dribbles are classified as challenges by one observer and not the other. Table 6.1(b) and (c) show an example of validation of the automated algorithm. It is known that there are 20 dribbles and the Is_Challenge function inspects the data relating to each

Table 6.1 Format of validation results (fictitious data)

**(a) Observer 1 v Observer 2**

| Observer 1 | | Observer 2 | |
| --- | --- | --- | --- |
| | Challenge | Not | Total |
| Challenge | 7 | 1 | 8 |
| Not | 2 | 10 | 12 |
| Total | 9 | 11 | 20 |

$P_0 = 0.85$
$P_C = 0.51$
$\kappa = 0.69$

**(b) Observer 1 v Algorithm**

| Observer 1 | | Automated algorithm | |
| --- | --- | --- | --- |
| | Challenge | Not | Total |
| Challenge | 6 | 2 | 8 |
| Not | 3 | 9 | 12 |
| Total | 9 | 11 | 20 |

$P_0 = 0.75$
$P_C = 0.51$
$\kappa = 0.49$

**(c) Observer 2 v Algorithm**

| Observer 2 | | Automated algorithm | |
| --- | --- | --- | --- |
| | Challenge | Not | Total |
| Challenge | 6 | 3 | 9 |
| Not | 3 | 8 | 11 |
| Total | 9 | 11 | 20 |

$P_0 = 0.70$
$P_C = 0.51$
$\kappa = 0.39$

of these classifying each as a challenge or not. The automated algorithm will have known loopholes and limitations and the computer will not be able to exercise the discretion and expertise of experienced human observers. This means that the method used by the human observers is different from that applied by the algorithm. Thus we are validating the algorithm against an alternative approach rather than doing a reliability study. We typically have greater levels of agreement between two human observers than between a human observer and the automated algorithm. The kappa values in Table 6.1(b) and (c) are interpreted as moderate and fair strengths of agreement respectively which may seem unsatisfactory. However, five or six disagreements between human and automated methods out of 20 cases may be expected and developers are encouraged to state the reasons for any disagreements that might be entirely understandable. Indeed, some such disagreements between human observation and the algorithm may be expected to the extent that higher values for strength of agreement might be too good to be true! O'Donoghue and Robinson (2009) did a validation study for cutting movements identified by an automated algorithm using the approach described here. The two human observers achieved a good strength of agreement while each human observer did not exceed a moderate strength of agreement with the automated algorithm. A complicating issue in the validation study done by O'Donoghue and Robinson (2009) was that the number of cases to be classified was unknown. This meant that as well as having values for each type of cutting movement, the validation study needed to consider where one method concluded a cutting movement occurred but another didn't. In the current example, we at least know the number of dribbles performed in the match according to the match event data.

## FURTHER AREAS FOR ANALYSING PLAYER TRACKING DATA

The current chapter has used the example of challenging in soccer to show how player tracking data can be analysed to provide tactical information to coaches and players. Numerical information about such tactical events can be provided but, more importantly, the algorithms locate the times of these events within matches allowing relevant video sequences to be accessed in a flexible manner. There are other areas identified earlier in this chapter that have been discussed within soccer coaching literature. Offensive soccer tactics with the potential to be analysed using player tracking and supporting match event data include:

1  creating space (Bangsbo and Peitersen, 2004:19–29);
2  approach runs, runs from the back;
3  wall passes (Bangsbo and Peitersen, 2004: 41–5);
4  overlaps (Bangsbo and Peitersen, 2004: 53–7; Hughes, 1994: 45–9), decoy runs and wide runs to the outside of the player dribbling the ball which can create depth and width for the attacking team;
5  change of tempo when in possession (Bangsbo and Peitersen, 2004: 155–9);
6  penetration (Bangsbo and Peitersen, 2004: 167–70) and beating the offside trap.

# 138

Defensive soccer tactics also offer areas for exploiting player tracking data. A leading textbook on defensive tactics in soccer (Bangsbo and Peitersen, 2002) identifies various areas including:

1   retreating (Bangsbo and Peitersen, 2002: 7);
2   marking distance (Bangsbo and Peitersen, 2002: 8);
3   forcing the opponent's direction (Bangsbo and Peitersen, 2002: 55–9);
4   man-to-man, zonal or combination cover (Bangsbo and Peitersen, 2002: 71–146);
5   team defensive depth, preventing free space behind the defence (Bangsbo and Peitersen, 2002: 147–9);
6   using the off-side trap (Bangsbo and Peitersen, 2002: 191–4).

There are some aspects of play that might be better being identified by match analysis personnel rather than an automated algorithm. For example, takeovers (Bangsbo and Peitersen, 2004: 67–72) are where the player initially dribbling the ball plays it to a teammate travelling towards him from the opposite direction and then the receiving player continues in the opposite direction. This changes the direction in which the ball is travelling. This could be in parallel or perpendicular to the opposition goal line. In deciding whether to create an automated system to analyse such an aspect, the developers need to consider the potential validity of such an algorithm, analysts data entry loads if the given event is to be entered manually as well as how many matches are to be analysed over the lifetime of the system. The greater the use of the algorithm, the easier it is to justify the cost of developing it.

Other aspects of play have been discussed without the quality of supporting data that player tracking systems offer. This may have led to misperceptions about these aspects of play. For example, Tenga *et al.* (2009) classified balance of the defence during opposing team possessions according to Olsen's (1981) principles. A fully balanced defence includes pressure, backup and cover. However, exploratory analysis of player tracking data by O'Donoghue (2011) has shown that the state of each one of these elements varies within possessions. For example, in a 10 second possession the opposing defence may switch from cover only, to cover and backup, to backup only and then none of the elements. These changes can happen very rapidly due to player movements during attacks. Therefore, some areas of soccer tactics need to be thoroughly investigated using player tracking data to give a fuller understanding of patterns and summary values associated with different types of tactics with differing outcomes.

## SUMMARY

The research done using player tracking data to date has not achieved the full potential offered by the data. This chapter proposes the combined use of match event data as well as player tracking data during the analysis of tactical aspects of movement. The approach consists of 5 stages: (a) selection of an aspect of play to be analysed; (b) operationalising this aspect; (c) specifying what the algorithm will do; (d) designing and implementing the algorithm; and (e) validating the algorithm. There are tactical events that might be recognised by expert human observation of match video in a more efficient and valid way than by using an automated algorithm. Therefore, the viability of any automated process for analysing player tracking data needs to be considered in terms of usefulness of the process, the number of matches it will be applied to and the development cost.

# CHAPTER 7

## MATLAB

### INTRODUCTION

Matlab is a computer programming language that can be used for data processing and visualisation. The language is supplied within a supporting environment with debugging tools and toolkits for different types of processing such as neural networks. Matlab is particularly powerful for processing large tables of data (arrays and matrices). The language has operators that can be efficiently applied to entire matrices as well as the conditional and iteration statements that are found in many other programming languages. In this chapter we will illustrate Matlab using three examples. The first two examples process player tracking data of the kind discussed in Chapter 6. The third example is a simulation study used to predict the outcome of the 2014 FIFA World Cup.

### ALGORITHMS AND DATA STRUCTURES

In sports performance analysis, Matlab is typically used to process large volumes of sports performance data in ways that would be awkward in standard spreadsheet and statistical analysis packages. Typically, we start with a large volume of data that needs to be processed in order to provide higher-level summary outputs. For example, we may analyse player tracking data to determine the times at which soccer players are in an offside position. These times could then be used to tag events in a match video that followed the on-the-ball action rather than the fixed camera video used to determine the player trajectories. Another example is that we may have

141

criteria for identifying where players perform different types of cutting movement and wish to determine the number of each type of cutting movement performed by each player. Matlab can be used in command mode or we can use a stored program. In command mode, we simply enter statements into the command area of the Matlab interface, creating new variables to be processed by further commands. This can be very efficient for ad hoc processing of data where conditional control and iteration of commands are not needed. Where a more complex task will be performed on more than one occasion, it is better to create a program and save it as an M-file script that can be loaded and executed any time in the future.

The basic philosophy of programming in sports performance analysis applications is to apply a 'pipeline' of procedures to gradually reduce the input data to the summary output data that are required. The procedures may be invoked by an overall controlling program, which means that the program code will be distributed over several M-file scripts. These may be arranged into an elaborate hierarchy of three or more levels of M-file scripts. As the overall program processes data, local data structures should be used to store intermediate results. This is very useful for isolating problems (bugs) in the program during its development. The raw data to be used can be loaded from external data files with the summary results appearing in tables, which can be pasted into spreadsheets and statistical analysis packages for further processing if necessary.

**THE INTERFACE**

Matlab will be stored on computers in different ways; it may be accessed through an icon on the desktop of the computer or through the programs menu or in an applications folder. Many universities will use many different application systems on their computers and so will arrange these in folders. For example at Cardiff Metropolitan University, students would look in the Applications folder, then the Sport folder within this and then the Performance Analysis folder where Matlab has been placed. The top-left hand side of the Matlab interface shows the directories that have been accessed recently while in the bottom left there is the command history. The area to the right is the command window, which shows the commands used and displays any result. These may be individual data processing commands or simply the names of any M-file scripts that have been executed.

142

There is a 'Workspace' tab where we can still see a command window, but this also shows a list of variables that we may wish to examine. These include our input data structures, intermediate data structures and variables as well as any output data structures. When we click on a variable or data structure that we are interested in, its value(s) appear in the array editor at the top right of the interface. This allows us to identify where any errors may have been made during the programming of early program versions. Syntax errors occur where the user has typed a command into an M-file script using the language incorrectly. The computer will not be able to understand such commands and thus will not be able to execute them. A statement may be syntactically correct but have semantic errors. For example, a correctly written assignment statement may be trying to assign a character string to a numerical variable. When syntax or semantic errors are made, the Matlab package halts the execution of the program, highlighting where the error occurred. This diagnostic information is very useful when correcting programs. Logical errors occur where the program is syntactically and semantically correct, has executed, but has produced incorrect results. These errors are much more difficult to detect and the computer cannot identify a logical error for us. The computer simply executes the instructions it is given without question and cannot know what we intended to do. Determining where logical errors have been made requires us to analyse intermediate results using the array editor area of the interface.

When executing a program in the command window, we need to state the name of the M-file script. If we include the folder where the program is stored in the known paths for Matlab, then we do not need to specify the full path of the file every time we execute it. We add a folder to the known folders by going to the **File** menu and selecting **Set Path**, choosing the **Add Folder** option and then selecting the folder of interest.

## CONSTANTS, VALUES AND VARIABLES

### Types

This chapter focuses on processing numerical data. However, Matlab supports other data types such as Boolean (logical) data, characters and character strings. Boolean variables use 1 and 0 to represent True and False respectively. Character strings can be expressed in single quotes, for example 'Brazil'. There are different types of numerical data types including integers and floating point numbers. We can specify the type of integer on the creation of a variable. For example, the following statement assigns the value 127 to an 8 bit integer, n.

    n = int8(127).

An 8 bit integer is ultimately represented by 8 binary digits (bits) the first bit of which is the sign bit. Therefore, the values are restricted to −128 to +127. We can also have 16, 32 and 64-bit integers. Where our values are cardinal numbers (whole numbers starting at zero without the need for a sign bit), we can represent a greater magnitude of number with the same number of bits. For example, if n were initialised as follows, it could take any value from 0 to 255 even though we give it an initial value of 127.

    n = unit8(127)

Real numbers are represented as single precision or double precision floating point numbers. Double precision floating point numbers are represented in 64 bits allowing values ranging from −1.79769e+308 to 1.79769e+308 to be represented. The 'e+308' means that the number to the left of the 'e' character is multiplied by $10^{308}$ or the decimal point is shifted 308 places to the right. The precision of this type also allows positive and negative numbers with small magnitudes to be represented, for example 2.22507e−308 shifts the decimal point 308 places to the left. This is the default type in Matlab but it is possible to specify that real numbers are represented as single precision floating point numbers if we wish to. Single precision floating point numbers are represented in 32 bits and so do not have the range or precision of double precision floating point numbers.

Character strings can be assigned to variables by specifying them in single quotes, for example:

    Team_name = 'Brazil';

Character strings can be processed using various string manipulation functions supplied by Matlab including 'strcat' which joins strings together and 'length' which returns the number of characters in a string.

# 144

## Variable names

In MatLab, a variable is used to represent a data item (such as a single number) or data structure (such as a table/matrix of numbers). A variable name can be up to 31 characters in length starting with a letter and then containing any combination of letters, digits and underscores. For example:

Table
M
M2
League_Table

## Matrices

An array is a table of values; this could be one dimensional, two dimensional or multi-dimensional. Consider the following command where A is the name of a two-dimensional array of values. The values assigned to this matrix are listed in square brackets to the right of the equal sign.

A = [16 3; 10 11; 7 12; 4 14]

This generates a matrix which has four rows and two columns.

A =
```
16    3
10    11
7     12
4     14
```

Subscripts are used in parentheses to address rows, columns or individual elements of matrices when we need to refer to these within commands. Some examples for our matrix A are:

A(2,1) = 10

A(1:3,1) =
```
16
10
7
```

```
A(:,1) =
      16
      10
       7
       4

A(3,:) =
       7      12

sum(A)
      37      40
```

Matrices can be constructed from existing matrices using concatenation (or joining). If we wished to create a matrix B that placed A on top of itself (i.e. eight rows and two columns), we would use the following command:

    B = [A;A]

This gives the following values to B.

```
B =
      16       3
      10      11
       7      12
       4      14
      16       3
      10      11
       7      12
       4      14
```

If, on the other hand, we wished to create a matrix B that was made up of two copies of A beside each other, we would use the following command:

    B = [A A]

This creates the following matrix of four rows and four columns.

B =

```
16    3    16    3
10   11    10   11
 7   12     7   12
 4   14     4   14
```

Rows and columns can be deleted but it is not possible to delete a sub-matrix from the middle of a matrix as the resulting structure must still be a matrix of some form. The following command deletes the third row from A:

A(3,:) = [ ]

Resulting in the following matrix of three rows and two columns

A =

```
16    3
10   11
 4   14
```

We could then use the following to delete the first column of A:

A(:,1) = [ ]

This leaves a as a matrix of three rows and one column.

A =   3
      11
      14

## NxN matrices

There are additional functions and processes that apply to square matrices. Consider the 3 × 3 matrix, B.

B = [3 2 13; 5 11 8; 15 14 4]
B =

```
 3     2    13
 5    11     8
15    14     4
```

We can create a single-column matrix formed of the top-left to bottom-right diagonal values of B.

diag(B) =
3
11
4

The sum command can be applied to any matrices but here it is used to specifically determine the sum of the values on the top-left to bottom-right diagonal of the square matrix B.

sum(diag(B)) = 18

B' is a transposed version of B:

B' =
| 3 | 5 | 15 |
| 2 | 11 | 14 |
| 13 | 8 | 4 |

## Generating matrices

We have already seen how matrices can be created by simply listing their values in square brackets. However, some matrices are large and creating them in this way can be cumbersome. Therefore, Matlab provides alternative ways of initialising matrices. Matrices can be initialised using zeros, ones, random numbers or even normally distributed random numbers. The following is used to set up a 3 × 3 matrix of zeros, M:

M = zeros(3,3)
M =
| 0 | 0 | 0 |
| 0 | 0 | 0 |
| 0 | 0 | 0 |

Alternatively, M could be initialised to a 3 × 3 matrix of containing the value 1 in each cell:

148

M = ones(3,3)

M =

| 1 | 1 | 1 |
|---|---|---|
| 1 | 1 | 1 |
| 1 | 1 | 1 |

When a matrix is multiplied by a numerical value, such as 7, every value within the matrix is multiplied by that value. This allows us to initialise M to being a 3 × 3 matrix containing 7 in each cell:

M = 7*ones(3,3)

M =

| 7 | 7 | 7 |
|---|---|---|
| 7 | 7 | 7 |
| 7 | 7 | 7 |

The following command initialises M to a 3 × 3 matrix of random numbers whose values are greater than or equal to 0 and less than 1.

M = rand(3,3)

M =

| 0.9501 | 0.4860 | 0.4565 |
|--------|--------|--------|
| 0.2311 | 0.8913 | 0.0185 |
| 0.6068 | 0.7621 | 0.8214 |

If the same 9 random numbers are generated, each time we execute our Matlab program, we can use the following command to set an initial random number using the real-time clock.

rand('state', sum(100*clock))

**Structures**

Sometimes the columns of data structures represent different components within rows that we would like to name. For example, a league table may have columns for team name, games played, wins, draws, losses, goals for, goals against, goal difference and points. It would be more convenient for programmers to refer to these columns as such rather than having to remember that column 5 contains games lost for example. Structures in Matlab are used for representing data with named fields. In the case of a league table, we would have an array of structures. For example, we may have a pool of 4 teams which can be set up as follows:

```
Team(1).Name = 'Brazil';
Team(2).Name = 'Croatia';
Team(3).Name = 'Mexico';
Team(4).Name = 'Cameroon';
for i = 1:4
  Team(i).Played = 0;
  Team(i).Won = 0;
  Team(i).Drawn = 0;
  Team(i).Lost = 0;
  Team(i).Goals_for = 0;
  Team(i).Goals_against = 0;
  Team(i).Goal_diff = 0;
  Team(i).Points = 0;
end
```

It is possible to have arrays within structures within arrays, etc. Therefore, a key design step in Matlab is how to represent the input and intermediate data we are processing as well as the information to be presented as output.

## BASIC STATEMENTS

### Assignment statements

In describing the initialisation of variables, we have already seen examples of the assignment statement that is used to initialise or change the value of a variable. The assignment statement takes the form:

Variable_name = expression

# 150

The expression on the right hand side of the equals symbol must be one that can be evaluated to a value of the same type and structure as the variable to the left of the equals symbol. For example, if the variable is numeric, then the expression must be evaluated to a numerical value. If the variable name identifies a matrix of a given structure, then the expression must evaluate to a matrix of the same structure. The expression on the right hand side could simply be a constant, for example:

```
i = 2
j = 3
```

These two commands set the values of i and j to 2 and 3 respectively.

We could assign the current value of a variable to another variable, for example the following command evaluates the current value of j (which is 3) and assigns it to the variable k.

```
k = j
```

The expression could be some numeric expression in terms of variables and constants, for example the following will assign the value 6 to the variable k:

```
k = i + j + 1
```

## Arithmetic operators and precedence

Table 7.1 shows the basic arithmetic operators used in Matlab. These are similar to the symbols used for arithmetic operators in most programming languages.

Table 7.1 Basic arithmetic operators

| Operator | Meaning | Example | Effect |
|----------|---------|---------|--------|
| + | Addition | k = 2 + 3 | k = 5 |
| − | Subtraction | k = 2 − 3 | k = -1 |
| * | Multiplication | k = 2 * 3 | k = 6 |
| / | Division | k = 2 / 3 | k = 0.6667 |
| ^ | Power | k = 2 ^ 3 | k = 8 |

Operators are applied in descending order of precedence (priority) with operators of the same precedence level being applied from left to right. Parentheses (round brackets) have the highest priority and can be used to over-ride the priority of other operators. Power has the second highest precedence. Multiplication and division are at the third level of precedence with addition and subtraction having the lowest precedence. Consider, the following expression being assigned to k where i and j are 2 and 3 respectively:

$$k = (i + j) \wedge 2 + i * 4 - j / 3$$

First, the sub-expression in parentheses is evaluated, (i + j) giving 5 leaving the following still to be computed:

$$k = 5 \wedge 2 + i * 4 - j / 3$$

The power operator is the highest priority, so 5 ^ 2 is evaluated to 25, leaving

$$k = 25 + i * 4 - j / 3$$

Multiplication and division are then applied from left to right, leaving the following to be evaluated:

$$k = 25 + 8 - 1$$

Finally, the addition and subtraction operators are applied from left to right giving a value of 32, which is assigned to k.

**Loading data from files**

Zeros, ones and random numbers can be too restrictive for some applications where specific data are needed. For example, the first two example programs used in this chapter need time-motion data from a particular match. The third example requires specific data about the draw for the FIFA World Cup 2014. Matrices can be loaded from tab delimited text files that can be created using Microsoft Excel. Once the data are entered into Excel in the correct format, the spreadsheet can be saved as a .CSV file (comma separated value file) or a text file. This can then be

152

loaded into Matlab using the following type of command where we know the absolute location of the file (in this case the file is called 'mymatrix.csv' and is in the 'matlab' folder on the 'H' drive).

> Load H:\matlab\mymatrix.csv

Alternatively, the file could exist in one of the directories whose path is known to Matlab, allowing us to simply specify the file name containing the data without specifying the full path.

> Load mymatrix.csv

## Using semi colons

Using a semi colon (;) at the end of an assignment statement will prevent the variable from being displayed in the command area of the interface when the sub-routines and functions are being executed. This may be useful where the variable is repeatedly updated within iteration statements (such as nested 'for' / 'while' loops) and we wish to speed up the execution of the routine.

## CONDITIONAL STATEMENTS

The statements of a Matlab program are executed in order unless the program code explicitly states otherwise. Sometimes we want more than a sequence of instructions that are executed one after the other. The normal order of statement execution is changed using program control structures such as conditional statements and iteration statements. The 'if' statement can be used to specify whether some inner statements are executed or not. The 'if' statement takes the following form:

```
if <Boolean condition>
    <Statement 1>;
    <Statement 2>;
    .
    .
    <Statement n>;
end
```

In this arbitrary example, statements 1 to n are only executed if the Boolean expression holds. For example, we may wish to avoid dividing by zero, so we could use the following:

```
if j ~= 0
   k = i / j;
end
```

The comparison operator '~=' is the not equal to operator. The 'if' statement can also include an else part. This allows one set of statements to be executed if some condition holds and some alternative set of statements to be executed if the condition does not hold. Consider the following to determine the outcome of a match (1 is win, 2 is loss) using a random number.

```
Score=rand(1)
if Score<0.5
   Result=1
else
   Result=2
end
```

The 'if' statement here uses '<' which is another comparison operator. 'Score<0.5' will be evaluated to True or False (the two Boolean values). If it is true, the statement after the 'if' will be executed, otherwise the statement after the 'else' will be executed. There are other comparison operators that are listed in Table 7.2. Note that '==' should not be confused with '=' that is used in assignment statements. The '==' comparison operator essentially asks if two expressions evaluate to the same

Table 7.2 Basic comparison operators (in the examples i = 2 and j = 3)

| Operator | Meaning | Example | Truth of example |
|----------|---------|---------|------------------|
| < | Less than | i < j | True |
| > | Greater than | i > j | False |
| == | Equal to | i == j | False |
| ~= | Not equal to | i ~= j | True |
| <= | Less than or equal to | i <= j | True |
| >= | Greater than or equal to | i >= j | False |

# 154

value while '=' means becomes equal to. This is why the assignment statement below makes sense:

j = j + 1

We know that j cannot equal itself plus 1. But we have not used '==' we have used '=' so we are saying evaluate j + 1 and assign the result to j.

We can also use an 'elseif' part of an 'if' statement whether we use an 'else' part or not. Imagine that we want to simulate a sports result where there is a 0.4 probability of a win (outcome 1), a 0.4 probability of a loss (outcome 2) and a 0.2 probability of a draw (outcome 0). This can be achieved using the following 'if' statement:

```
Score=rand(1)
if Score<0.4
    Result=1
elseif Score>0.6
    Result=2
else
    Result=0
end
```

Sometimes we wish to use AND or OR conditions together when forming Boolean expressions. When doing so we should beware that the AND and OR Boolean operators (&& and || respectively) have a higher precedence than the comparison operators shown in Table 7.2. Therefore, parentheses may have to be used as illustrated in this following example to test if a value is between 4 and 7 inclusive:

```
if (4 <= i) && (i <=7)
    k = 1
end
```

## ITERATION STATEMENTS

The 'for' statement is used to execute a sequence of instructions a predetermined number of times. The following 'for' statement computes the sum of the first 10 positive integers. This particular 'for' statement executes the inner statement (Total = total + i) varying i from 1 to 10 in steps of 1.

```
Total = 0;
for i=1:10
    Total = Total + i;
end
```

The 'while' statement differs from the 'for' statement in that it repeats some inner statement(s) while some condition holds. It tests some condition and if the condition holds, the inner statements are executed and then the condition is tested again. This continues until the condition is evaluated to False. The following 'while' statement determines the number of positive integers starting at 1 that need to be added together to exceed 100. The 'while' statement leaves n with a value that is 1 greater than the last value of n that was added to Total. Therefore, we take 1 away from n after the 'file' statement has completed.

```
n=1
Total = 0
while Total <= 100
    Total = Total + n;
    n = n + 1;
end
n = n - 1;
```

## EXAMPLE 1: DISTANCE COVERED IN DIFFERENT SPEED RANGES

### Purpose

The purpose of this example is to determine the distribution of match time among different speed zones that players move at. The data come from a single match period of 45 minutes and 26s and there are 22 players. The program examines player locations that have been recorded every 1s and determines the percentage of time spent in the following speed zones:

- $0$ m.s$^{-1}$
- Faster than $0$ m.s$^{-1}$ but slower than $2$ m.s$^{-1}$

- Equal to or faster than 2 m.s$^{-1}$ but slower than 4 m.s$^{-1}$
- Equal to or faster than 4 m.s$^{-1}$ but slower than 5.5 m.s$^{-1}$
- Equal to or faster than 5.5 m.s$^{-1}$ but slower than 7 m.s$^{-1}$
- Equal to or faster than 7 m.s$^{-1}$

## Data file

The data file txy.csv is a comma separated value file that contains 2736 rows of data; one row of data for each second where player locations were recorded. The structure of the file is shown in Figure 7.1. There are 45 columns: the first column represents the match time in seconds, columns 2 to 23 are 22 columns representing the locations of the home team players (Team A) while columns 24 to 45 are 22 columns representing the locations of away team players (Team B). Columns 2 and 3 represent the X and Y coordinates of the home team's goalkeeper. Figure 7.2 shows the dimensions of the football pitch. X represents the back to forward location on the pitch with −57m being Team A's own goal line, 0m being the halfway line and +57m being Team B's goal line. The value of Y ranges from −40 to +40 with −40 representing the left side line for Team A and +40 representing the right side line for Team A. The coordinates (0,0) represent the centre circle. Columns 4 and 5 are the X and Y coordinates of the next Team A player with columns 22 and 23 representing the X and Y coordinates of the 11th Team A player. Columns 24 to 45 are arranged in the same way for Team B with columns 24 and 25 representing the X and Y coordinates of their goalkeeper and columns 44 and 45 representing the X and Y coordinates of their 11th player.

| Time |  Team A |  |  |  |  | Team B |  |  |  |  |
|------|--------|--------|--------|--------|--------|--------|--------|--------|--------|--------|
|  | Keeper |  |  | Player 11 |  | Keeper |  |  | Player 11 |  |
| Col 1 | Col 2 | Col 3 |  | Col 22 | Col 23 | Col 24 | Col 25 |  | Col 44 | Col 45 |
| 1 |  |  | ......... |  |  |  |  | ......... |  |  |
| 2 |  |  |  |  |  |  |  |  |  |  |
| 3 |  |  |  |  |  |  |  |  |  |  |
| . |  |  |  |  |  |  |  |  |  |  |
| . |  |  |  |  |  |  |  |  |  |  |
| . |  |  |  |  |  |  |  |  |  |  |
| 2736 |  |  |  |  |  |  |  |  |  |  |

Figure 7.1 Structure of the txy.csv file

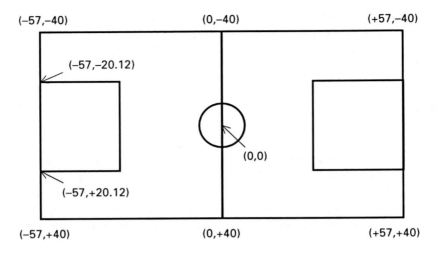

Figure 7.2 Dimensions of the football pitch

**Program design and implementation**

The program is made up of four phases:

1 initialisation of variables;
2 determine distance covered in each second of the match by each player;
3 determine the number of seconds spent in each speed range by each player;
4 convert the number of seconds in each speed zone to a percentage of match time for all players.

The code is shown below this paragraph. Note that any line starting with a '%' character is a comment that is not executed. Comments are included to document the program for the purposes of clarity and maintenance. Comments should mediate between the problem and program domains rather than merely repeating statements in English. The first 5 lines initialise variables. The data are loaded from the file and are stored in a matrix txy that has 2736 rows and 45 columns. An intermediate matrix 'Distance' is used to determine the distance travelled in each second of

158

the match by each player. This requires 2736 rows and 22 columns. This could have been done in 2735 rows because the distance is from the previous time point and the first row of data in the file do not have any previous rows of locations where players have travelled from. The decision to stick with 2736 rows was so that each row of the 'Distance' matrix would correspond to a row of the txy matrix. There are 6 speed zones and so the matrix 'Percent' has rows (one for each speed zone) and 22 columns (one for each player).

```
01| load txy.csv;
02| % declare variables
03| n=2736;
04| Distance = zeros(n,22);
05| Percent = zeros(6,22);
06| for i = 2:n
07|     % work out distance covered and speed since last time point
08|     % do this for each player
09|     for j = 1:22
10|         x1 = txy(i−1,j*2);
11|         y1 = txy(i−1,j*2+1);
12|         x2 = txy(i,j*2);
13|         y2 = txy(i,j*2+1);
14|         % from Pythagoras
15|         Distance(i,j) = sqrt(((x1-x2)^2)+((y1-y2)^2));
16|     end
17| end
18| % now we want to add up volume of time spent in different
    speed zones
19| for i=2:n
20|     for j=1:22
21|         if Distance(i,j) == 0
22|             Percent(1,j) = Percent(1,j)+1;
23|         elseif Distance(i,j) < 2
24|             Percent(2,j) = Percent(2,j)+1;
25|         elseif Distance(i,j) < 4
26|             Percent(3,j) = Percent(3,j)+1;
27|         elseif Distance(i,j) < 5.5
28|             Percent(4,j) = Percent(4,j)+1;
29|         elseif Distance(i,j) < 7
30|             Percent(5,j) = Percent(5,j)+1;
```

```
31 |          else
32 |                    Percent(6,j) = Percent(6,j)+1;
33 |          end
34 |   end
35 | end
36 | % Now turn these into percentages
37 | for k=1:6
38 |    for j=1:22
39 |            Percent(k,j) = 100*Percent(k,j)/(n−1);
40 |    end
41 | end
```

Lines 6 to 17 perform the second stage and determine the distance travelled by each player during each second of the match. Each of these distances is an estimate assuming that the player has travelled in a straight line between the two recorded locations at a time point and previous time point. The outer 'for' loop ('for i = 2:n') deals with each time point in turn from 2s into the match to 2736s. It starts at 2s because there was no previous time point that was travelled from at 1s. The inner loop ('for j = 1:22') deals with the 22 players. Within these two nested loops we need to retrieve the location travelled from (x1,y1) and travelled to (x2,y2) by player j at time i. This is done in lines 10 to 13. The location travelled from is in row i−1 of the txy matrix and the location travelled to is in row i. Consider player 3 (j = 3) whose X and Y coordinates are stored in the columns 6 and 7 respectively. The expression j*2 gives the column for the X coordinate and the expression j*2+1 gives the column for the Y coordinate. Lines 10 to 13 use the i and j indexes to retrieve the correct values for each player at each point in time. Line 15 applies Pythagoras' Theory to estimate the distance travelled and store it in the 'Distance' matrix.

Lines 18 to 35 perform the third step by inspecting each value in the 'Distance' array and updating the 'Percent' array. Note that because our time periods are 1s intervals, the value for distance in any time interval is also the mean speed in that 1s interval. If a player travelled 4.7m in 1s, the mean speed was 4.7m.s$^{-1}$. We have 6 options and so a structured 'if' statement with 4 'elseif' parts and an 'else' part is used (lines 21 to 33). Consider where we ask if the speed is less than 5.5m.s$^{-1}$ (line 27). We do not actually need to explicitly state that the speed must be greater than or equal to 4m.s$^{-1}$ and less than 5.5mm.s$^{-1}$ for the player to be in the

# 160

4th of our 6 speed zones. The previous 'if' and 'elseif' parts have already asked if the player was travelling at 0m.s⁻¹, less than 2m.s⁻¹ or less than 4m.s⁻¹. Matlab would not be inspecting the condition 'Distance(i,j) < 5.5' unless the previously specified conditions had already been evaluated as False.

On completion of the two nested loops (lines 19 to 35) we will have the total number of seconds spent in each speed zone by each player stored in the 'Percent' matrix. The purpose of the fourth phase of the program is to determine the percentage of time spent in each speed zone. Lines 36 and 41 transform the volume of time for each player in each speed zone to a percentage of the 2735s of match time. Note that there are 2736 time points and so technically there are only 2735 one second intervals between these. Therefore, we produce the percentage by multiplying each value in 'Percent' by 100 and dividing by $(n-1)$. This is done in line 39.

## EXAMPLE 2: BALANCE OF DEFENCE IN SOCCER

### Purpose

Olsen (1981) described a soccer defence as being balanced if it applied pressure, backup and cover. Figure 7.3 illustrates the modified version of Olsen's definitions used by O'Donoghue (2011). Olsen described a defender as applying pressure if they were within 1.5m of the opposing ball carrier and goal side of the ball carrier. Defenders providing backup would be within 5m of the opposing ball carrier while being goal side. Any other goal side defenders are described as providing cover. The defence is fully balanced when it applies pressure, backup and cover. When O'Donoghue (2011) applied these definitions to Prozone data, he discovered that representing 'goal side' as a triangle formed by the opposing ball carrier's location and the goal posts was too restrictive and there were surprisingly few occasions where pressure, backup or cover were applied. Therefore, O'Donoghue (2011) used the back corners of the penalty area to complete the triangle with the opposing ball carrier as shown in Figure 7.3.

The purpose of this program is to determine how often pressure, backup and cover as well as any combination of these are applied to the forward most opponent, when the opposing team is in possession. There are two files of input data. The first is the same 'txy.csv' file containing the

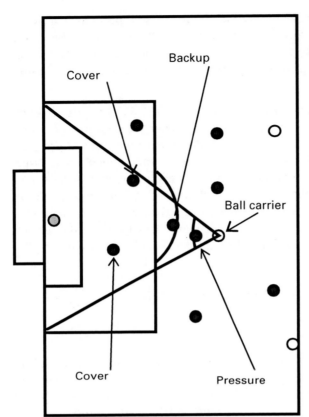

**Figure 7.3** A balanced defence applying pressure, backup and cover

Note (black dots for defenders and grey dot for goalkeeper)

locations of all 22 players that was used in the previous example. The second file is called 'poss.csv' and contains data about the possessions that occurred in the first half. The team, outcome, start time, end time and duration of each possession are stored in this second file.

The output that we want is the percentage of time that the team spends exerting pressure, backup, cover and any combination of these on the forward most opposing player. The different combinations are illustrated in the Venn diagram shown in Figure 7.4. The values given are the times for the whole first half of a match reported by O'Donoghue (2011). This example has the advantage of only considering times when the opposing team has possession of the ball.

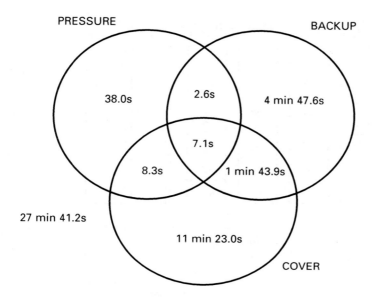

PRESSURE

BACKUP

38.0s

2.6s

4 min 47.6s

7.1s

8.3s

1 min 43.9s

27 min 41.2s

11 min 23.0s

COVER

Figure 7.4 Distribution of match time

## Design

With an example like this, we need to think out a way of processing the data and map out the criteria for recognising pressure, backup and cover. Figure 7.5 shows the data structures involved, which give an indication of the processes needed. The first thing to be done is to determine the forward most opponent and the location of the forward most opponent for each 1s period of the first half. Once this is done, we can use the data about the forward most opponent to determine whether or not each player is in the triangle shown in Figure 7.3. This requires a 2736 × 10 matrix, because there are 2736 time points and 10 outfield players on our team. Pythagoras' Theory is used to determine the distance between each player to the forward most opponent. This also requires a 2736 × 10 matrix to be populated. The next step inspects these two 2736 × 10 arrays to determine the number of players providing pressure, backup and cover at any of the 1s periods. This is used to create the 2736 × 8 matrix called 'venn_time'. The 8 columns are used to represent the following states of the defence:

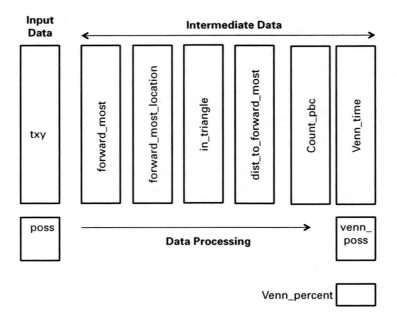

Figure 7.5 Data structures used during the analysis of defensive balance

1   no pressure, backup or cover applied;
2   cover only;
3   backup only;
4   cover and backup;
5   pressure only;
6   pressure and cover;
7   pressure and backup;
8   pressure, backup and cover (fully balanced defence).

Once this has been determined for the whole first half, the poss file can be inspected to determine the number of seconds the defence is in each of these states when the opposing team has the ball. This is then used to determine the percentage of time the defence is in each of the eight different states.

The M-file script Main.m is an overall control program that invokes procedures to gradually reduce the data to the form we wish to output. There are only five statements in Main.m:

164

1   initialisation;
2   find_forward_most;
3   check_triangle;
4   check_balance;
5   process_possessions;

The Initialise.m M-file script loads the two comma separated value files and initialises the intermediate matrices to containing zeros. Note, in line 7, we have specified that there are exactly 107 possessions.

```
01| % Load the external data files
02| load poss.csv;
03| load txy.csv
04| % Note the number of timed data points n
05| n = 2736;
06| % Note the number of possessions
07| npos = 107;
08| % Set up the intermediate pipeline of data structures
09| forward_most = zeros(n,1);
10| forward_most_location = zeros(n,2);
11| in_triangle = zeros(n,10);
12| dist_to_forward_most = zeros(n,10);
13| count_pbc = zeros(n,3);
14| venn_time = zeros(n,8);
15| venn_poss = zeros(npos,8);
16| venn_percent = zeros(1,8);
```

The M-file script Find_forward_most.m is shown below. The outer 'for' loop applies lines 2 to 14 to each time point where data have been gathered. At each point in time the forward most player starts off as the 2nd opponent to exclude their goalkeeper (lines 3 and 4). Remember from the previous example, that the opposing players' coordinates are stored in columns 24 to 45 of the txy matrix. Therefore, the expression 22+2*j will give us the X coordinate for the jth opposing player. The 'for' loop from line 6 to line 11 then checks each of the other opponents in turn. Our team plays from left to right so if the opponent's X coordinate is less than the lowest found so far then this opposing player becomes the new forward most opponent. On completing this inner loop, the X and Y coordinate of the forward most player are stored in forward_most_location (lines 13 and 14).

```
01|  for i = 1:n
02|     % Forward most so far is Team B's first outfield player
03|     forward_most(i,1) = 2;
04|     forward_most_x = txy(i,22+2*2);
05|     % check if remaining players in turn are further forward
06|     for j=3:11
07|        if txy(i,22+2*j) < forward_most_x
08|           forward_most(i,1) = j;
09|           forward_most_x = txy(i,22+2*j);
10|        end
11|     end
12|     % and save the forward most location
13|     forward_most_location(i,1) = txy(i,22+2*forward_most(i,1));
14|     forward_most_location(i,2) = txy(i,23+2*forward_most(i,1));
15|  end
```

The Check_triangle.m M-file script is the most challenging and we need to sit down with pen and paper and devise a way to work out *exactly* if a player is in the triangle formed by the forward most opponent and the back corners of the penalty area. Figure 7.6 shows the geometry of this problem. We know the forward most opponent's location (x_opp, y_opp) and we know the defender's location (x_plr, y_plr). We use an imaginary vertical line where x = x_plr. For the defender to be within the triangle, they must be between the points where two of the lines of the triangle intersect the line x = x_plr. We can work out the horizontal distance from the goal line to the defender (x_plr + 57) and from the goal line to the opponent (x_opp + 57). The value of y_min can be calculated by scaling the vertical distance from −20.12 to y_opp by the ratio of the horizontal distance to the player and the opponent. This can also be done for y_max. This scaling is shown in lines 11 and 12 of the Check_triangle.m M-file script.

The outer 'for' loop (lines 1 to 22) ensures that we check each time point while the inner 'for' loop (lines 6 to 21) ensures that we check each outfield player. The location of the opponent (x_opp, y_opp) is retrieved from the forward_most_location matrix in lines 3 and 4. The locations of our players are stored in columns 2 to 23 of the txy matrix. The column of the jth player's X coordinate is 2*j while the jth player's Y coordinate is in column 2*j+1. This location is retrieved from the txy matrix in lines 7 and 8. Once y_min and y_max are determined, we simply need to work

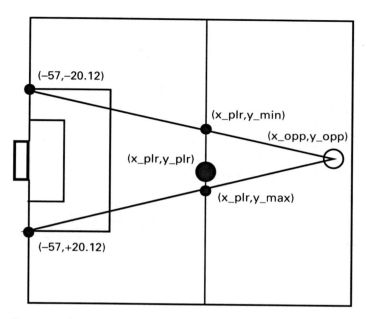

(−57,−20.12)

(x_plr,y_min)

(x_opp,y_opp)

(x_plr,y_plr)

(x_plr,y_max)

(−57,+20.12)

**Figure 7.6** Determining if defender is in the triangle formed by forward most opponent and the back corners of the penalty area

Note: (Defender is black dot, opponent is white dot)

out if the player's Y coordinate (y_plr) is in between these and if so we record this in the in_triangle matrix. This is done in line 14 where y_min < y_plr < y_max is implemented by AND-ing two conditions together '(y_min < y_plr)&&(y_plr < y_max)'. Note in line 20 that column j−1 of in_triangle is used to record this for player j. This is because we only record details for the ten outfield players.

```
01 |  for i=1:n
02 |    % look up location of forward most opponent
03 |    x_opp = forward_most_location(i,1);
04 |    y_opp = forward_most_location(i,2);
05 |    % check if any players are in the triangle
06 |    for j = 2:11
07 |      x_plr = txy(i, 2*j);
08 |      y_plr = txy(i, 2*j+1);
09 |      if x_plr < x_opp
```

```
10 |          % determine min and max y values in triangle for
             player's x
11 |          y_min = −20.12 + (y_opp+20.12)*(−57 − x_plr)/(−57 −
             x_opp);
12 |          y_max = 20.12 − (20.12-y_opp)*(−57 − x_plr)/(−57 −
             x_opp);
13 |          % is player's y between y_min and y_max
14 |          if (y_min < y_plr) && (y_plr < y_max)
15 |              %yes the player is in the triangle
16 |              in_triangle(i,j−1)=1;
17 |          end
18 |      end
19 |      % Save the distance to the forward most player
20 |      dist_to_forward_most(i,j−1)  =  sqrt(((x_plr-x_opp)^2)+
         ((y_plr-y_opp)^2));
21 |  end
22 | end
```

The payoff for the effort made in determining if each of our players is in
the triangle formed by the forward most opponent and the back corners
of the penalty area comes when we write the Check_balance.m M-file
script that is shown below. As usual there is an outer loop (lines 1 to 56)
to make sure the processing is applied to each time point. Lines 3 to 16
check if each player is in the triangle and if any are, then they apply pressure, backup or cover depending on how far they are away from the
forward most opponent. Lines 17 to 55 implement three levels of 'if-else'
statements to determine which combination of 0, 1, 2 or all three of pressure, backup and cover applies at the current time point. These lines of
code simply represent a decision tree as nested 'if' statements.

```
01 | for i = 1:n
02 |   % check if player provides pressure, backup or cover
03 |   for j = 2:11
04 |       if in_triangle(i,j−1) == 1
05 |           if dist_to_forward_most(i,j−1) < 1.5
06 |               % Pressure
07 |               count_pbc(i,1)=count_pbc(i,1)+1;
08 |           elseif dist_to_forward_most(i,j−1) < 5
09 |               % Backup
10 |               count_pbc(i,2)=count_pbc(i,2)+1;
```

```
11 |          else
12 |              % Cover
13 |              count_pbc(i,3)=count_pbc(i,3)+1;
14 |          end
15 |      end
16 |  end
17 |  % at this time what does the venn diagram look like
18 |  if count_pbc(i,1) > 0
19 |      if count_pbc(i,2) > 0
20 |          if count_pbc(i,3) > 0
21 |              % Pressure, Backup and Cover
22 |              venn_time(i,8) = 1;
23 |          else
24 |              % Pressure and Backup
25 |              venn_time(i,7) = 1;
26 |          end
27 |      else
28 |          if count_pbc(i,3) > 0
29 |              % Pressure and Cover
30 |              venn_time(i,6) = 1;
31 |          else
32 |              % Pressure
33 |              venn_time(i,5) = 1;
34 |          end
35 |      end
36 |  else
38 |      if count_pbc(i,2) > 0
39 |          if count_pbc(i,3) > 0
40 |              % Backup and Cover
41 |              venn_time(i,4) = 1;
42 |          else
43 |              % Backup
44 |              venn_time(i,3) = 1;
45 |          end
46 |      else
47 |          if count_pbc(i,3) > 0
48 |              % Cover
49 |              venn_time(i,2) = 1;
50 |          else
51 |              % Nothing
```

```
52 |              venn_time(i,1) = 1;
53 |           end
54 |        end
55 |    end
56 | end
```

Now that all of the processing has been completed for each time point, we access the poss matrix within the Process_possessions.m M-file script to determine the percentage of time the defence is in each of the 8 balance states (Figure 7.6) during opposition possessions. The outer 'for' loop (lines 3 to 18) deals with the possessions with the 'if' statement (lines 5 to 17) ensuring that we only deal with opposition possessions; the first column of the poss matrix represents the team in possession. The start and end time of any possession where Team B (Team 2 in poss) is in possession is retrieved (lines 7 and 8) and used in the 'for' loop (lines 11 to 16) that processes an individual possession. The inner 'for' loop (lines 12 to 15) adds up the time spent in each of the eight balance states. Once this is completed, line 20 uses the total time the opponents have been in possession to convert the eight values within the venn_percent matrix to percentage defending time values rather than total time in seconds.

```
01 | % Initialise total time for Team B's possessions
02 | Team_B_Poss_Time = 0;
03 | for k=1:npos
04 |    % Only deal with Team B's possessions
05 |    if poss(k,1) == 2
06 |        % Get start and end time of possession
07 |        start_time = poss(k,2);
08 |        end_time = poss(k,3);
09 |        Team_B_Poss_Time = Team_B_Poss_Time + end_time +
              1 - start_time;
10 |        % Count the balance states within the possession
11 |        for i = start_time:end_time
12 |            for m=1:8
13 |                venn_poss(k,m)=venn_poss(k,m)+venn_time(i,m);
14 |                venn_percent(1,m)=venn_percent(1,m)+venn_time
                      (i,m);
15 |            end
16 |        end
17 |    end
```

```
18 |  end
19 |  % Complete the percentages
20 |  venn_percent = 100*venn_percent / Team_B_Poss_Time;
```

## EXAMPLE 3: SIMULATION OF 2014 FIFA WORLD CUP

Simulation represents the real world as a system with a model of inter-relations between variables within the system (Martin, 2011). This section of the chapter describes the use of Matlab to perform a stochastic simulation of the 2014 FIFA World Cup to be played in Brazil. Stochastic simulations represent random chance, which is important given the unpredictable nature of soccer matches. Simulations are not just used to make predictions but also to develop understanding of systems and explanations for issues arising from the predictions.

SPSS and Matlab were used to produce a prediction of the World Cup. A set of 207 soccer matches from previous international tournaments played since 2006 was used to produce a model for match outcome. The match outcome variable is the difference in goals scored between the higher ranked team and the lower ranked team within the match according to the FIFA world rankings. Linear regression was applied to the previous match data using 3 independent variables:

- difference in FIFA World ranking points between the two teams;
- difference in distance from the capital city of the team to the capital city of the host nation between the two teams;
- difference in the number of days since the previous match played within the tournament. A default value of zero was used if it was the teams' first match within the tournament.

Only the first of these independent variables was a significant predictor of goal difference between the two teams in the match. However, the full regression model shown in Equation 7.1 was used as the underlying model of the simulation system. This model suggests that every 424 FIFA world ranking points a team is ahead of the opposition is worth a goal. However, there is little evidence of home advantage. If a team travelled 10,000 km further than their opponents to a tournament, it would only be worth 0.143 goals to the opponents. Having an extra recovery day over the opponents from the last matches played by the two teams is actually detrimental to performance according to this model. If a team had five days from the previous match and the opposing team had only four days recovery, the extra recovery day the team had would be worth 0.107 goals to the opponents.

$$
\begin{aligned}
\text{Goal Diff} = \ & {-}0.0483 \\
& + 0.00236 \ \text{Ranking Points Diff} \\
& - 0.0000143 \ \text{Distance Travelled Diff} \\
& - 0.107 \ \text{Recovery Days Diff}
\end{aligned}
\tag{7.1}
$$

The scatter plots for goal difference plotted against each independent variable showed considerable variability about the lines of best fit. The residual values for the data had a standard deviation of 1.890. This was used within the simulator in order to ensure that any random variation about the expected result was evidenced by the spread of values evidenced from previous international soccer matches.

The 32 teams contesting the 2014 FIFA World Cup were known at the time this chapter was written. The FIFA world ranking points posted on the official FIFA website on 13 March 2014 (www.fifa.org, accessed 14 March 2014) were initialised within the package along with the giant circle distance from each country's capital city and Brasilia, the capital city of Brazil. The schedule of matches within the tournament was known and so differences in recovery days to be experienced by pairs of teams contesting matches was also represented by the system. The simulator was implemented as a hierarchy of Matlab program files as shown in Figure 7.7. The simulator initialised variables, simulated the tournament 20,000 times and then reported progression statistics for the 32 teams within the simulated tournaments. The DrawGroups component was fixed and used the official draw for the 2014 tournament. The groups were played by simulating the six matches within each group, determining the group table and the two teams qualifying from the group.

The Matlab file simulating a group match is shown below. The variables gt1 and gt2 are numbers between 1 and 4 representing the teams within the current group, gr. These allow the teams' identities (numbers between 1 and 32) to be looked up from 8 × 4 Group matrix. These identities are used to look up ranking points and distances travelled in lines 8 and 9 respectively. If a match has a predicted goal difference between −0.5 and +0.5 then it is considered to be a draw. Lines 10 and 11 set up these threshold values for a loss and a win respectively. RecAdv is the number

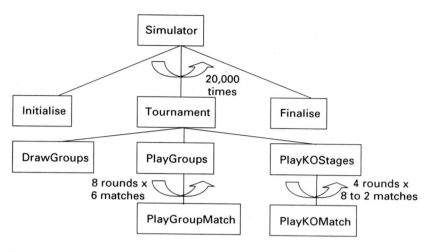

Figure 7.7 Structure of the World Cup simulator

of additional recovery days team1 has over team2; this is passed into the PlayGroupMatch subroutine as a global variable. Lines 12 to 16 apply the regression equation to determine the expected goal difference between the two teams, exp, using the regression equation. This is used to bias the simulation to ensure higher ranked teams have a greater chance of winning simulated matches than lower ranked teams. Line 17 simulates the throwing of a 100 sided dice. Line 18 uses this to look up a z-score within a standard normal distribution curve, multiplying the z score by the known standard deviation of 1.890 for the residuals in previous soccer match outcomes. This could cause the team to win by more than expected, lose or draw depending on the random number that is produced. Lines 19 to 22 update the group table recognising the two teams have played a game (column 1 of Table) and the goal difference within the match is applied to column 7 of Table. Lines 23 and 27 determine whether the match was a win, draw or loss for team 1 within the match comparing goaldiff to the threshold values for a win and a loss. If the team won then their number of wins (column 2 of Table) is incremented by 1 and their points (column 8 of Table) is raised by 3 while team2's losses (column 4 of Table) is incremented by 1. The opposite happens if team2 has won the match. If the match was drawn, both teams have their draw count (column 3 of Table) incremented by 1 and their points (column 8 of Table) are raised by 1 point each.

```
01 | % PlayGroupMatch
02 | % Group gr
03 | % Team 1 gt1
04 | % Team 2 gt2
05 | % RecAdv is number of extra recovery days for team 1
06 | team1 = Group(gr,gt1);
07 | team2 = Group(gr,gt2);
08 | rankpdiff = Team(team1,2) − Team(team2,2);
09 | distdiff = Team(team1,3) − Team(team2,3);
10 | win_threshold = 0.5;
11 | lose_threshold = −0.5;
12 | if rankpdiff > 0
13 |    exp = −0.0483 + 0.00236*rankpdiff − 0.0000143*distdiff −
         0.107*RecAdv;
14 | else
15 |    exp = 0.0483 + 0.00236*rankpdiff − 0.0000143*distdiff −
         0.107*RecAdv;
16 | end
17 | dice = round(rand(1)*99+1);
18 | goaldiff = exp + 1.890*NormDist(dice,1);
19 | Table(gt1,1)=Table(gt1,1)+1;
20 | Table(gt1,7)=Table(gt1,7)+goaldiff;
21 | Table(gt2,1)=Table(gt2,1)+1;
22 | Table(gt2,7)=Table(gt2,7)-goaldiff;
23 | if goaldiff > win_threshold
24 |    Table(gt1,2)=Table(gt1,2)+1;
25 |    Table(gt2,4)=Table(gt2,4)+1;
26 |    Table(gt1,8)=Table(gt1,8)+3;
27 | elseif goaldiff < lose_threshold
28 |    Table(gt2,2)=Table(gt2,2)+1;
29 |    Table(gt1,4)=Table(gt1,4)+1;
30 |    Table(gt2,8)=Table(gt2,8)+3;
31 | else
32 |    Table(gt2,3)=Table(gt2,3)+1;
33 |    Table(gt1,3)=Table(gt1,3)+1;
34 |    Table(gt1,8)=Table(gt1,8)+1;
35 |    Table(gt2,8)=Table(gt2,8)+1;
36 | end
```

The Matlab code for a knockout match is similar except there are no draws and teams are no longer in groups of four. The threshold value is simply set to zero. Therefore, a goaldiff value of greater than +0.5 represents a team winning in normal time, while a value between 0.0 and +0.5 means that the team would have won after extra time or a penalty shootout. Similarly, a goaldiff value of less than −0.5 represents a team losing in normal time, while a value between −0.5 and 0.0 means that the team would have lost after extra time or a penalty shootout. The winning team is forwarded to the appropriate location in the knockout structure. The simulator revealed that Spain had the highest chance of winning the 2014 FIFA World Cup having won 22.2% of the simulated tournaments as shown in Figure 7.8. However, this is not an overall majority of the simulated tournaments and there is a 77.8% chance that the tournament will be won by somebody else. There is a 9.7% chance that the tournament will be won by a team outside the highest ranked 16 teams competing in it. It's wide open!

The advantages of using simulation are that it is economic, controllable and safe (Martin, 2011). However, Martin has also discussed disadvantages of simulations. Human behaviour is very complex and simulations

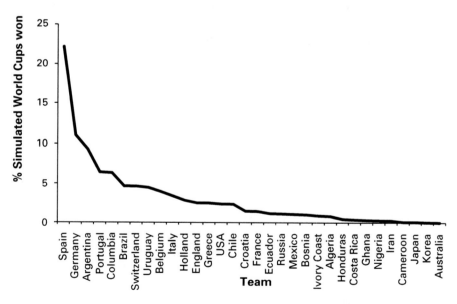

**Figure 7.8** Probability of each team winning the 2014 FIFA World Cup according to the simulation system

matlab

such as the one described in the current chapter may over-simplify real world behaviour. The simulator is based on a regression model of match score in terms of three well-defined parameters. There are numerous relevant variables that have not been included in the model. These include players not available due to injury, discipline, travel within the tournament between matches, cultural factors, climate, playing tactics and varying club commitments of players prior to the tournament.

## SUMMARY

This chapter has shown how Matlab can be used to process large volumes of sports performance data, specifically player tracking data. A key skill in using any programming language is problem solving. How can we represent the data? What processing strategy should we use? How can we process the data to reduce it in the way that we need? What language facilities will help us to do this? Matlab provides facilities for data storage and retrieval as well as program control structures for iteration and conditional control. These can be used as building blocks in the construction of algorithms. Program files can invoke other program files allowing systems to be developed as hierarchical structures of algorithmic components. This chapter has used examples of Matlab for data processing as well as a processor-intensive simulation system.

# CHAPTER 8

## STATISTICAL ANALYSIS

### INTRODUCTION

This chapter is concerned with statistical analysis of sports performance data. The chapter covers descriptive statistics as well as inferential statistics. Descriptive statistics summarise performances using chosen performance variables. Typically this is done using a reductive approach where multiple performance data are analysed to determine an average performance. Sample statistics such as frequencies, modes, medians, means and standard deviations are used to describe samples. Relationships between variables are described using correlation coefficients. Inferential statistics are used to compare samples in terms of performance variables. These samples could be performances of different classes of performer or performances by the same performers under different conditions (for example at home and away). There are many different ways of investigating the same area of sports performance. This chapter describes four alternative ways of analysing tennis data depending on whether point, match, player performance within a match or player performance over multiple matches is used as the unit of analysis. Once the descriptive statistics have provided average values to represent the samples, inferential statistics can be used to determine if any differences between those samples are significant. The inferential procedures used in performance analysis are typically non-parametric techniques as the data rarely satisfy the assumptions of parametric procedures. The chapter uses Statistics Package for Social Sciences (SPSS) (SPSS, An IBM company, Amarouk, NY) as an example statistics package to illustrate the process of statistical analysis of sports performance data. Statistical analysis is relatively straightforward once data are organised into a structure permitting this analysis. Therefore, the first half of this chapter is concerned with the data preparation tasks that occur prior to data analysis.

## WHAT TEST TO USE WHEN?

Many statistics textbooks have outlined which statistical test to do in which situation (Diamantopoulos and Schlegelmilch, 1997: 174; Vincent, 1999: inside back cover; Hinton, 2004: inside front cover; Salkind, 2004: 180–1; Fallowfield *et al.*, 2005: 153, 182, 217, 262; O'Donoghue, 2010: 180; O'Donoghue, 2012: 127–32). The current chapter covers non-parametric techniques. However, there are occasions where parametric tests can be justified. Where sports performance data satisfy the assumptions of normality and homogeneity of variances, parametric statistics should be used because they are more powerful than their non-parametric equivalents. Where interactive effects need to be tested, parametric statistics permit this but the non-parametric alternatives covered in the chapter don't. An interactive effect is where the combination of two or more independent variables has an influence on a dependent variable beyond the effects of any individual independent variables. For example, some performance indicators in a sport may be significantly influenced by the interaction of venue and match period. The difference between the performance indicator value in the first and second halves of a soccer match, for example, might be different when playing at home than when playing away from home. The other situation where parametric procedures may be justified is when we have small volumes of data. Imagine a situation where we are comparing performance in the first and second half in a sample of 7 soccer matches. There are only so many arrangements of rankings that can be made, restricting the number of different p values that can result from a non-parametric test (the Wilcoxon signed ranks test in this situation). This makes it more difficult to achieve a significant difference than if a parametric test was used (a paired samples t-test in this situation). Therefore, to give the investigation some chance of finding a significant difference, the researcher might choose to use a parametric test, acknowledging the fact that the data do not satisfy one or more assumptions of the test. In selecting a non-parametric statistical procedure, we need to understand the purpose of our study, the variables involved and the nature of the samples. Figure 8.1 is a decision tree that can be used to decide on a procedure.

178

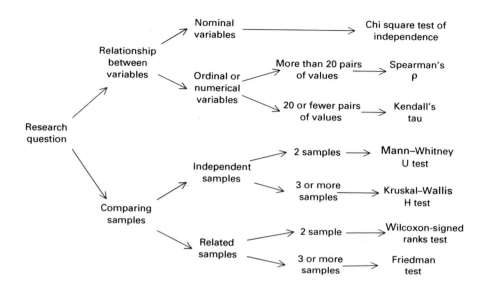

Figure 8.1 Decision tree for selecting a statistical test

## DATA PREPARATION

### The data

This chapter uses the example of Grand Slam tennis data taken from the official websites of the four Grand Slam tennis tournaments played in 2012 (Australian Open, French Open, Wimbledon, US Open). The Excel spreadsheet 'Grand-Slam-2012.xls' contains the data used in this chapter. The sheet 'Performances' contains the data that were gathered from the websites. There were potentially 2032 player performances (2 genders × 4 tournaments × 127 matches × 2 player performances per match). However, some matches were not completed due to disqualification of a player, retirement of a player or the match being a walkover. The 1966 player performances from the 983 completed singles matches within the 'Grand-Slam-2012.xls' spreadsheet are included in the 'Performances' sheet. There is a row for each player performance, hence two rows per match. There is a single row of column headings at the top of the sheet. There are columns for the following variables:

- Column A: Match Identification Number
- Column B: Gender (1 = Female, 2 = Male)
- Column C: Tournament (1 = Australian Open, 2 = French Open, 3 = Wimbledon, 4 = US Open)
- Column D: Round (1 to 7; 5 = quarter final, 6 = semi final, 7 = final)
- Column E: Outcome (1 = won, 2 = lost)
- Column F: Player 52-week ranking for singles at the time of the tournament
- Column G: Player name
- Column H: Opponent 52-week ranking for singles at the time of the tournament
- Column I: Opponent name
- Column J: Frequency of points won on 1st serve
- Column K: Frequency of 1st serve points played
- Column L: Frequency of points won on 2nd serve
- Column M: Frequency of 2nd serve points played
- Column N: Percentage of points where 1st serve is in
- Column O: Percentage of points won when 1st serve is in
- Column P: Percentage of points won when 2nd serve is required
- Column Q: Opponent percentage of points where 1st serve is in
- Column R: Opponent percentage of points won when 1st serve is in
- Column S: Opponent percentage of points won when 2nd serve is required

The last three columns may look like redundant copies of other players' data but when we are profiling we may wish to consider a player's receiving performance (as characterised by what the opponent was able to do on serve) as well as the serving performance.

## Basic rules

There are some basic rules that we must adhere to when preparing data for analysis in SPSS. In this example, the data are prepared in Microsoft Excel. These rules are listed below:

- there must be one and only one row of headings;
- there must be a row for each case (participant, performance or whatever unit of analysis is being used);

180

- there must be a column for each variable (including repeated measures of variables).

When we are preparing spreadsheets of data to be uploaded into SPSS, we must bear these rules in mind while creating the spreadsheet. It is more efficient to prepare the spreadsheet in the correct format in the first place than have to spend hours restructuring the data later.

The last point about repeated measures of variables comes from an important philosophical distinction between conceptual variables and the variables that are included in SPSS. Imagine an investigation to analyse the influence of gender on the percentage of points where the first serve is in. We have a conceptual independent variable (gender) and a conceptual dependent variable (percentage of points where the first serve is in) that we hypothesise depended, to a certain extent, on gender. We have a column for the independent variable in this sheet and a single column for the dependent variable. The independent variable (gender) is a grouping variable that distinguishes different sets of player performances; those within women's singles matches and those within men's singles matches. Now consider an investigation where we wish to analyse the effect of service (first or second) on the percentage of points won. Conceptually, we have a single independent variable (service) and a single dependent variable (percentage of points won). We have hypothesised that the percentage of points won, to a certain extent, depends on service. The way in which the SPSS data sheet is organised means that we can only have one row of data for each case. Therefore, we need two repeated measures of the conceptual dependent variable; percentage of points won when the first serve is in and percentage of points won when the second serve is in. We actually will not have a column in the data sheet for the variable service. This is because it is not a grouping variable; all players play points where the first serve is in and when a second serve is required. Any situation where we have a variable measured at different times, or under different conditions, for the same cases, we have repeated measures of some conceptual variable. The SPSS data sheet needs a column for each repeated measure of the variable. So for example, if we had the shooting percentage of basketball players in each quarter, we would have 4 repeated measures of the shooting percentage variable; one for each quarter.

You will have noticed that numerical codes have been used for gender and tournament. There are three reasons for this. First, it is easier to type in 1 and 2 than 'Female' and 'Male'. Second, if we did try to type in 'Female' and type in 'female', SPSS would consider these to be different values. The third reason for using numerical codes is that some analyses in SPSS actually require grouping variables to be numerically coded. These include two of the non-parametric tests that will be covered in the current chapter. Where a user has typed in value names, such as 'Female' and 'Male', these can be automatically recoded within a numerical variable in SPSS.

## Planning the analysis

Before data are collected, the researcher should have considered the research problem and specified a precise research question that is testable. This will have helped identify the data to be collected. The null hypotheses to be tested in the current example are:

- gender has no influence on the percentage of points where the first serve is in, the percentage of points won when the first serve is in or the percentage of points won when a second serve is required;
- tournament has no influence on the percentage of points where the first serve is in, the percentage of points won when the first serve is in or the percentage of points won when a second serve is required;
- gender has no influence on the proportion of matches that are upsets;
- tournament has no influence on the proportion of matches that are upsets;
- the percentage of points where the first serve is in is similar between the winning and losing players within matches;
- there is no difference between the winning and losing players within matches for the percentage of points won when the first serve is in or when a second serve is required.

There are variations on these null hypotheses that can be tested. For example, we could examine the effect of gender on variables within separate tournaments. Similarly, we could examine the effect of tournament on variables for women's singles and men's singles separately. The performances of winning and losing players could be compared for each of the eight game types (2 genders × 4 tournaments) separately. We could analyse these different effects using player performance as the unit of analysis (n = 1966). Alternatively, we could average winning and losing

182

player's values within a match to have match as the unit of analysis (n = 983). This can be criticised for artificially reducing the natural variability in sports performance data. Some have used individual match events (such as points) as the unit of analysis. We have 180,488 points played in the 983 matches. These could be analysed as nominal variables but this approach has been criticised because there is excessive non-independence in the data (O'Donoghue *et al.*, 2012). A further way of analysing the data is to use player as the unit of analysis. We may be concerned that different players succeed at different tournaments and, therefore, any differences between the tournaments are more to do with the players contesting the later rounds of those tournaments than the tournaments themselves. We could insist on the same players being used to compare the four tournaments by having average values for the variables of interest within each tournament for a set of players who have completed a sufficient number of matches at each tournament. This involves using player as the unit of analysis. As we will see later in this chapter, using player as the unit of analysis and applying a criteria for inclusion in the study of at least three performances within each tournament, we will only have six female and nine male players. There is an argument to be made that if a player gets to the final, and hence plays seven matches at a tournament, it is because the player's game is suited to the requirements of the tournament. Therefore, including more performances for this player than those eliminated in earlier rounds is producing more realistic results.

Once the data have been collected, we can consider how the data can be processed into the correct form to allow statistical analysis in the chosen statistics package. This chapter will use four different units of analyses to illustrate different statistical procedures in SPSS and Excel; these are summarised in Table 8.1. This chapter will now explain how the data can be pre-processed into the different formats shown in Table 8.1.

**Performance as the unit of analysis**

The data were originally entered into the 'Performances' sheet of the spreadsheet, meaning that no further pre-processing was necessary if using player performance as the unit of analysis. The data can now be loaded into SPSS. On entering the SPSS package, go to the **File** menu, choose **Open** and then choose **Data**. In this chapter, the notation **File** →

Table 8.1 Analyses of a dependent variable (DV) using alternative units of analysis

| Unit of analysis | Data sheet | Hypotheses to be tested | Test |
|---|---|---|---|
| Point | Summing | Gender effect on DV | Chi square |
| | | Tournament effect on DV | Chi square |
| Player performance | Performances | Gender effect on DV | Mann–Whitney U |
| | | Tournament effect on DV | Kruskal–Wallis H |
| | | Relation between variables | Spearman's ρ |
| Match | Matches | Player (winner v loser) on DV | Wilcoxon |
| | | Gender effect on proportion of upsets | Chi square |
| | | Tournament effect on proportion of upsets | Chi square |
| Player | Tournament comparison | Tournament effect on proportion of upsets | Friedman |

Open → Data is used to represent the navigation through menus and submenus. In the popup window that appears, you need to select 'File of type'; choose Excel. Go to the folder where the Excel file exists and choose the file 'Grand-Slam-2012.xls'. Click on the 'Open' button. This will give you a choice of worksheets to open; choose 'Performances'. The data will now appear in the SPSS datasheet. Save this file as 'Performances'; it will have the '.SAV' extension (the file already exists in the material provided with the book). The 'Variable View' tab is used to allow us to change variables' types, number of decimal places used and to add value labels. The variables 'Gender', 'Tournament', 'Outcome' and 'Round' have 0 decimal places as they are numerically coded variables. 'Player Rank' and 'Opp Player Rank' are whole numbers and do not need any decimal places either. The Value column is used to provide value labels for any numerically coded variables. For example, Gender has the value labels 'Female' and 'Male' associated with the values 1 and 2. Once the value labels have been included for Tournament and

184

Outcome, the file is saved again. The process of loading the data into SPSS and defining the variables in SPSS is similar for the other SPSS files described in this chapter.

## Match as the unit of analysis

The original data in the 'Performances' sheet of the 'Grand-Slam-2012.xls' Excel file is processed to create the 'Matches' worksheet. This worksheet contains half of the rows that the 'Performances' sheet does; there is a row for each match. First, all of the data from the 'Performances' sheet is copied and pasted into the 'Matches' sheet. The data are then sorted on 'Outcome' and 'Match' as primary and secondary keys. If the functions evaluating percentages in the 'Performances' worksheet were still present then the data would actually be pasted into the 'Matches' worksheet using 'Paste Values'. This means that the percentage values will still persist in the 'Matches' worksheet when the frequency data that are no longer needed are deleted. The raw frequency variable columns J to M are deleted because we will only be analysing the percentage variables that address the fact that matches are of different lengths. The rows from 985 to 1967 are deleted because all of the data for winning and losing players' performances within each match are stored in the rows for the winning players and had been duplicated within the 'Performance' sheet. Now we have a single row for each match. The headings in row 1 are changed to reflect that these are specifically for the winning and losing players within matches rather than for the player and the opponent. Column P is a new column 'Upset', which takes the value 'Y' or 'N' depending on whether the match was an upset or not. An upset is where the match is won by the higher ranked player. The function shown in Figure 8.2 is used in the cell P2 to determine if the match in row 2 was an upset or not. This is copied and pasted into the remaining rows. This sheet is now ready to be loaded into SPSS where it is saved as 'Matches.SAV'.

| | ... | F | ... | H | ... | P |
|---|---|---|---|---|---|---|
| 1 | | Winner Rank | | Loser Rank | | Upset |
| 2 | | 1 | | 109 | | =IF(F2 > H2, "Y","N") |

Figure 8.2 Use of a conditional function to determine if a tennis match was an upset or not

## Player as unit of analysis

This analysis uses those players who have completed at least three matches in each of the four Grand Slam tennis tournaments in 2012. The mean values for the percentage of first serves that are in, percentage of points won when the first serve is in, percentage of points won when a second serve is required for the player and the opponent are included in the 'Tournament comparison' worksheet; this is 24 variables in total in addition to the players' names and genders. The process of producing this summary data from the original data in the 'Performances' worksheet is described. There are other ways in which the same result could be obtained. The important thing is to understand the required format of the resulting information and how functions and facilities of Excel can be used to process the data achieving this result.

The initial stage of the process is to determine the players who satisfy the criteria for inclusion which is to have completed in at least three matches at all four tournaments. This is done using a pivot table. The columns B to G of the original 'Performances' worksheet contain general tournament and match identification data. These columns are selected and **Insert →Pivot Table** is used to create a pivot table on a new worksheet which we call 'Frequency'. The columns B to G include tournament and player name which we need to cross-tabulate. The pivot table is set up by dragging 'Gender' and then 'Player Name' into the Rows area and 'Tournament' into the Columns area. 'Tournament' is then dragged into the Sum values area. We now see a cross-tabulation of players (grouped within the two gender categories) and tournaments showing the number of matches that each player played at each tournament. The whole pivot table is copied and the values pasted (**paste → values**) into the cells I3:O457 of the same worksheet so that we can work with values rather than the links in the pivot table that refer back to the 'Performances' sheet. The four columns J to M contain the frequency of matches players played at each tournament. A blank cell (rather than 0) represents where a player did not play any matches at a given tournament. Figure 8.3 illustrates how the IF function in the cell P2 determines whether or not the player in row 2 meets the criteria for inclusion. The player needs to have 4 values indicating that they have played matches in all four tournaments and the minimum value for match count at each tournament is greater than two. Column P is given the heading 'Included' and the values are 'Y' or 'N'. There are six women and nine men who satisfy the criteria for inclusion.

# 186

| | I | J | K | L | M | ... | P |
|---|---|---|---|---|---|---|---|
| 1 | Player | Aus | Fr | Wimb | US | | Include |
| 2 | Agnieszka Radwanska | 5 | 3 | 7 | 4 | | =IF((COUNT(J6:M6)=4)*AND(MIN(J6:M6)>2), "Y", "N") |

Figure 8.3 A conditional function to determine if a player has competed in three matches at each of the four Grand Slam tournaments or not

The next step is to determine the mean values for the different variables for each tournament. This involves creating a more ambitious pivot table than that in the 'Frequency' worksheet. Columns B to S in the 'Performances' worksheet are selected and then the pivot table is initiated using **Insert → Pivot** and asking for it to be placed in a new worksheet, which we name 'Player Tournament Means'. The variables 'Gender' and then 'Player Name' are dragged into the Row area. Tournament is dragged into the Column area. Now our six numerical variables of interest are dragged into the Sum Values area. These are:

- the percentage of points where the first serve is in;
- the percentage of points won when the first serve is in;
- the percentage of points won when a second serve is required;
- the percentage of points where the first serve is in for the opponent;
- the percentage of points won when the first serve is in for the opponent;
- the percentage of points won when a second serve is required for the opponent.

At the moment, we simply see counts of the number of values that there are. We need to click on the triangle to the right of each variable where it says 'Sum Values'. Choose 'Value field Settings' so that a popup window appears where we choose 'Average' rather than 'Count'. We now have four sets of six columns. We create a new worksheet 'Tournament comparison' where we copy the data from the 'Frequency' worksheet using paste values (**paste → values**). The values from the 'Player Tournament Means' worksheet are then copied and pasted (**paste → values**) into the 'Tournament comparison' worksheet beside the values we have already placed there. This is necessary to make sure that the names from 'Frequency' and 'Player Tournament Means' have been pasted into the same rows of the 'Tournament comparison' worksheet. This sheet is then sorted on 'Included' and 'Gender' as primary and secondary keys. The 15 players satisfying the criteria for inclusion are now in the final 15 rows of the worksheet and those players not included can be deleted. We only require 'Player name', 'Gender' and the four sets of six numerical variables. The remaining columns can be deleted. Finally, we tidy up the column headings using 'A_First In', 'A_Won1', 'A_Won2', 'A_Opp_First In', 'A_Opp_Won1', 'A_Opp_Won2' for the Australian Open, replacing 'A_' with 'F_', 'W_', 'U_' for the French Open, Wimbledon and the US Open respectively. The 'Replace All' facility comes in very handy here. These data can now be loaded into SPSS, reducing the number of decimal places and labelling the gender values in Variable View. The SPSS file is saved as 'Tournament Comparison.SAV'. The players included are listed below:

- Agnieszka Radwanska
- Ana Ivanovic
- Angelique Kerber
- Maria Sharapova
- Petra Kvitova
- Victoria Azarenka
- Andy Murray
- David Ferrer
- Janko Tipsarevic
- Juan Martin Del Potro
- Julien Benneteau
- Nicolas Almagro
- Novak Djokovic
- Richard Gasquet
- Roger Federer

**Point as unit of analysis**

When point is the unit of analysis, it is actually counter-productive to use SPSS if we can already produce cross tabulated frequencies. For SPSS to perform the chi square tests, we would need a row for each of the 180,488 points played. Instead, we can pre-process the data to allow the frequencies of interest to be analysed in Excel. The sheet 'Summing' is created using a pivot table from within the 'Performances' sheet.

The cells B to M in the 'Performances' worksheet are selected to include Gender, Tournament and the four frequency variables 'Points won on 1st

Serve', '1st serve points played', 'Points won on 2nd serve' and '2nd serve points played'. We use **Insert → Pivot Table** choosing to deposit the pivot table in a new work sheet, which we will call 'Summing'. 'Gender' and 'Tournament' are dragged into the Row area with our four frequency variables of interest being dragged into the Sum values area. For each numerical variable, we click on the triangle to the right of it and select Value field settings. Choose 'Sum' and click on OK and we now see the total frequency of points of each type in each tournament for women's and men's singles. These frequencies can now be used within chi square tests that will be described in the next section of the chapter.

## CHI SQUARE TESTS IN EXCEL

The chi square test of independence is illustrated using the percentage of points where the first serve is in. The purpose of the test is to determine if two categorical variables are independent of each other. For example, we have one variable 'Service', which indicates whether a point emanated from a first or second serve, and Tournament. If these two variables were completely independent, we would expect to see very similar percentages of points emanating from first serve at each tournament. The purpose of the chi square test of independence is to test if any differences between tournaments for the proportion of points emanating from first serve (and also from second serve) are statistically significant. The data from the 'Summing' sheet are copied, pasted and organised into the 'Chi Square for First Serve' sheet. The data are summarised in Table 8.2.

Table 8.2 Frequency of points where first serve was in and out at different tournaments (values in parentheses are percentages)

| Gender | Tournament | First serve in | Second serve required | Total |
|--------|-----------|----------------|-----------------------|-------|
| Women | Australian Open | 10037 (61.7) | 6234 (38.3) | 16271 |
| | French Open | 11404 (62.8) | 6745 (37.2) | 18149 |
| | Wimbledon | 11163 (63.4) | 6443 (36.6) | 17606 |
| | US Open | 9987 (60.6) | 6493 (39.4) | 16480 |
| | Total | 42591 (62.2) | 25915 (37.8) | 68506 |
| Men | Australian Open | 16218 (61.4) | 10199 (38.6) | 26417 |
| | French Open | 16872 (61.1) | 10745 (38.9) | 27617 |
| | Wimbledon | 18568 (63.6) | 10607 (36.4) | 29175 |
| | US Open | 16821 (58.5) | 11952 (41.5) | 28773 |
| | Total | 68479 (61.2) | 43503 (38.8) | 111982 |

Figure 8.4 shows a section of the 'Chi Square for First Serve In' worksheet, which performs the chi square test of independence. The observed frequencies shown in Table 8.2 are found in the cells B5:D16 of worksheet. Figure 8.4 only illustrates this for women's singles (rows 1 to 9). Figure 8.4 shows the values that are computed using the formulae in Figure 8.4. The spreadsheet is programmed to use the equation for chi square described by Vincent and Weir (2012: 272–7). Equation 8.1 gives us the chi squared value. This is determined in a number of steps in Excel: first the expected frequencies are determined, then the terms within the summation of equation (8.1) are determined and finally the sum of the terms is computed.

$$\chi^2 = \sum \frac{(Observed\ Frequency - Expected\ Frequency)^2}{Expected\ Frequency} \qquad (8.1)$$

| | A | B | C | D | ... | I | J | K | ... | M | N | ... | P | Q | R |
|---|---|---|---|---|---|---|---|---|---|---|---|---|---|---|---|
| 1 | | Observed | | | | Expected | | | | Calculation | | | Chi2 | DF | p |
| 2 | | | | | | | | | | | | | | | |
| 3 | | 1st In | 2nd req | Total | | 1st In | 2nd req | Total | | | | | | | |
| 4 | Female | | | | | | | | | | | | | | |
| 5 | Aus | 10037 | 6234 | 16271 | | =$D5*B$9/$D$9 | =$D5*C$9/$D$9 | =SUM(I5:J5) | | =POWER(B5-I5,2)/I5 | =POWER(C5-J5,2)/J5 | | =SUM(M5:N8) | 3 | =CHIDIST(P5,Q5) |
| 6 | French | 11404 | 6745 | 18149 | | =$D6*B$9/$D$9 | =$D6*C$9/$D$9 | =SUM(I6:J6) | | =POWER(B6-I6,2)/I6 | =POWER(C6-J6,2)/J6 | | | | |
| 7 | Wimb | 11163 | 6443 | 17606 | | =$D7*B$9/$D$9 | =$D7*C$9/$D$9 | =SUM(I7:J7) | | =POWER(B7-I7,2)/I7 | =POWER(C7-J7,2)/J7 | | | | |
| 8 | US | 9987 | 6493 | 16480 | | =$D8*B$9/$D$9 | =$D8*C$9/$D$9 | =SUM(I8:J8) | | =POWER(B8-I8,2)/I8 | =POWER(C8-J8,2)/J8 | | | | |
| 9 | Total | 42591 | 25915 | 68506 | | =SUM(I5:I8) | =SUM(J5:J8) | =SUM(I9:J9) | | | | | | | |

Figure 8.4 Performing a chi square test of independence in Microsoft Excel

| | A | B | C | D | ... | I | J | K | ... | M | N | ... | P | Q | R |
|---|---|---|---|---|---|---|---|---|---|---|---|---|---|---|---|
| 1 | | Observed | | | | Expected | | | | Calculation | | | Chi2 | DF | p |
| 2 | | | | | | | | | | | | | | | |
| 3 | | 1st In | 2nd req | Total | | 1st In | 2nd req | Total | | | | | | | |
| 4 | Female | | | | | | | | | | | | | | |
| 5 | Aus | 10037 | 6234 | 16271 | | 10115.9 | 6155.1 | 16271 | | 0.62 | 1.01 | | 33.7 | 3 | 2.29E-07 |
| 6 | French | 11404 | 6745 | 18149 | | 11283.5 | 6865.6 | 18149 | | 1.29 | 2.12 | | | | |
| 7 | Wimb | 11163 | 6443 | 17606 | | 10945.9 | 6660.1 | 17606 | | 4.31 | 7.08 | | | | |
| 8 | US | 9987 | 6493 | 16480 | | 10245.8 | 6234.2 | 16480 | | 6.54 | 10.74 | | | | |
| 9 | Total | 42591 | 25915 | 68506 | | 42591 | 25915 | 68506 | | | | | | | |

Figure 8.5 Performing a chi square test of independence in Microsoft Excel

190

The expected frequencies are determined using the total frequencies. For example, consider the effect of tournament on the proportion of first serves that are in during women's singles matches. There are 62.2% of points in women's singles where the first serve is in. If tournament has absolutely no effect on the percentage of points where the first serve is in, then we would expect this percentage of 62.2 to apply to each tournament individually. This is how our expected frequencies are computed. In the cells I5:J8, we actually use fractions, for example the expected frequency of points where the first serve is in at the Australian Open (women's singles) is 16271 × (42591 / 68506). For the cell I5 where this expected frequency is computed we type '=$D5*B$9/$D$9' as shown in Figure 8.4. Note the use of the '$' character for when referencing column D and row 9, which are where our totals are. These absolute references (rather than relative references) to cells mean that the cell I5 can be pasted into the remaining cells of I5:J9. The terms that are summed in Equation 8.2 are calculated in cells M5:N8. The cell M5 is the term for first serves at the Australian Open and uses the observed (B5) and expected (I5) frequencies for these values. The eight values in the cells M5:N8 are summed in the cell P5, which is the chi square value of 33.7. The number of degrees of freedom is the (rows – 1) × (columns – 1) which is 3 as shown in cell Q5. The CHIDIST function is used in cell R5 to calculate the p value using the chi square value and the degrees of freedom. This evaluates to a very low p value of 2.3E–07 or 0.00000023 because E–7 means the decimal place moves seven places to the left. For men's singles the decimal point is moved 35 places to the left (1.8E–35) giving a very small probability that the different proportions between the tournaments are down to chance/sampling error. The differences of note are the biggest differences to the overall gender proportions; this seems to be Wimbledon (lower percentage of first serves in than expected) and the US Open (greater percentage of first served in) in each gender.

The issue with this use of chi square is that there is non-independence in the data. It is as if we had 68,506 questionnaires from four groups of females who answered yes or no to some question. The issue here is that there are not 68,506 player performances and we have tricked chi square into thinking there are more data than there actually are.

**Exercise 8.1**

Use points as the unit of analysis to determine: (a) if the proportion of points won when the first serve is in is significantly influenced by tournament; and (b) if the proportion of points won when a second serve is required is significantly influenced by tournament. Perform these analyses for women's and men's singles separately.

## DATA ANALYSIS IN SPSS

### Chi Square test of independence

The chi square test of independence is used to test the null hypothesis that two categorical variables are independent of each other. Where the frequency distribution of one of those variables is proportionally similar for each value of the other variable, they are independent of each other. For example, if we consider the 983 tennis matches in our 'Matches' SPSS data sheet, we might ask if upsets are independent of gender. If we see a similar frequency profile of match outcomes between women's and men's singles then gender and match outcome will be independent. If, however, we see a much greater proportion of upsets for one gender than the other then there may be a significant association between gender and outcome.

Open the 'Match.SAV' file in SPSS. In the first analysis we will test whether gender and upsets are independent. The chi square test of independence is accessed through the statistics option when we cross-tabulate categorical variables. Use **Analyse → Descriptive Statistics → Crosstabs** to access the popup window to set up a crosstabulation. 'Gender' is transferred into Rows and 'Upset' is transferred into Columns. Click on **Cells** and, in the Cells popup window, tick the box to ask for percentages of rows. These are useful where we have a different number of women's and men's singles matches and it is not immediately obvious which has the greater proportion of upsets. The **Continue** button is used to get rid of the Cells popup window once we have checked the percentages we want. Click on **Statistics** and when the Statistics popup window appears, ask for Chi square by ticking it. Click on **Continue** to close the Statistics popup window and then click on **OK** in the Cross-tabulation popup window to execute the cross-tabulation and supplementary chi square test that we have requested. The output in Tables 8.3(a) and 8.3(b) appear: Table 8.3(a) shows the descriptive statistics while Table 8.3(b) shows the chi square results. The 149/496 (30.0%) of women's singles matches were upsets was greater than the 122/486 (25.1%) of men's singles matches. However, this is not significant ($\chi^2_1 = 3.0$, $p = 0.087$). The different bits of what has just been expressed in parentheses are now explained. The $\chi^2$ is the test statistic produced by the chi square test of independence. We have a 2×2 crosstabulation and so there is 1 degree of freedom (the 1 is subscripted). The number of degrees of freedom is given by the (rows − 1) × (columns − 1). The value of chi square is 2.995, which rounds to 3.0 as we are only using one decimal place for the test statistic. Anywhere we see 'Sig' in SPSS, it is actually referring to a p value, which is a probability of a Type I error. Given that probabilities have values between 0 and 1, this author

Table 8.3(a)  Crosstabulation output from SPSS

**Gender * Upset Crosstabulation**

|  |  |  | Upset N | Upset Y | Total |
|---|---|---|---|---|---|
| Gender | Female | Count | 347 | 149 | 496 |
|  |  | % within Gender | 70.0% | 30.0% | 100.0% |
|  | Male | Count | 364 | 122 | 486 |
|  |  | % within Gender | 74.9% | 25.1% | 100.0% |
| Total |  | Count | 711 | 271 | 982 |
|  |  | % within Gender | 72.4% | 27.6% | 100.0% |

Table 8.3(b)  Chi square output from SPSS

**Chi-square tests**

|  | Value | df | Asymp. Sig. (2-sided) | Exact Sig. (2-sided) | Exact Sig. (1-sided) |
|---|---|---|---|---|---|
| Pearson Chi-Square | 2.995[a] | 1 | .084 |  |  |
| Continuity Correction[b] | 2.753 | 1 | .097 |  |  |
| Likelihood Ratio | 2.999 | 1 | .083 |  |  |
| Fisher's Exact Test |  |  |  | .087 | .048 |
| N of Valid Cases | 982 |  |  |  |  |

Notes: a. 0 cells (0.0%) have expected count less than 5. The minimum expected count is 134.12.
    b. Computed only for a 2×2 table

expresses p values to 3 decimal places. Usually we would use the p value (Sig) from the Pearson's Chi Square row of results. However, when we have a 2 × 2 cross-tabulation, we use Fisher's Exact test (2 tailed). This gives a p value of 0.087, which is not significant where we count p values of less than 0.05 as significant. The 2 × 2 cross-tabulation has a better chance of yielding a significant result than larger cross-tabulations. Fisher's Exact test gives a slightly higher p value helping to reduce the chance of a Type I Error being made.

The previous example pooled all four tournaments together to analyse the association between gender and upsets. We might wish to look at this association between gender and match outcome for the four tournaments separately. This can be done by logically splitting the file into four partitions, one for each tournament, and then repeating the analysis we have just done. When the file is split, any analysis we do in SPSS is done for each partition of the file separately. We split the file on tournament using **Data → Split File**. Select 'Compare Groups', transfer 'Tournament into the 'Groups based on' area and click on OK. Now perform the cross-tabulation and supplementary chi square test exactly the same way as before and the output in Tables 8.4(a) and 8.4(b) are produced. The 48/126 (38.1%) of women's singles matches were upsets was significantly greater than the 26/122 (21.3%) of men's singles matches at the French Open ($\chi^2_1$ = 8.3, p = 0.005). There was no significant association between gender and upsets at any of the other three tournaments (p > 0.05). There is almost combined effect of gender and tournament here with more upsets in men's singles than women's singles at Wimbledon, while there are more upsets in women's singles than men's singles at all other tournaments.

### Exercise 8.2

Is the proportion of upsets influenced by tournament? Use a chi square test of independence and produce the necessary descriptive statistics for women's and men's single separately.

### The Mann–Whitney U test

The purpose of the Mann–Whitney U test is to compare two independent samples in terms of some variable that is measured on at least an

**Gender * Upset Crosstabulation**

| Tournament | | | | | Upset N | Upset Y | Total |
|---|---|---|---|---|---|---|---|
| Australian Open | Gender | Female | Count | | 87 | 36 | 123 |
| | | | % within gender | | 70.7% | 29.3% | 100.0% |
| | | Male | Count | | 92 | 26 | 118 |
| | | | % within gender | | 78.0% | 22.0% | 100.0% |
| | Total | | Count | | 179 | 62 | 241 |
| | | | % within gender | | 74.3% | 25.7% | 100.0% |
| French Open | Gender | Female | Count | | 78 | 48 | 126 |
| | | | % within gender | | 61.9% | 38.1% | 100.0% |
| | | Male | Count | | 96 | 26 | 122 |
| | | | % within gender | | 78.7% | 21.3% | 100.0% |
| | Total | | Count | | 174 | 74 | 248 |
| | | | % within gender | | 70.2% | 29.8% | 100.0% |
| Wimbledon | Gender | Female | Count | | 94 | 31 | 125 |
| | | | % within gender | | 75.2% | 24.8% | 100.0% |
| | | Male | Count | | 82 | 40 | 122 |
| | | | % within gender | | 67.2% | 32.8% | 100.0% |
| | Total | | Count | | 176 | 71 | 247 |
| | | | % within gender | | 71.3% | 28.7% | 100.0% |
| US Open | Gender | Female | Count | | 88 | 34 | 122 |
| | | | % within gender | | 72.1% | 27.9% | 100.0% |
| | | Male | Count | | 94 | 30 | 124 |
| | | | % within gender | | 75.8% | 24.2% | 100.0% |
| | Total | | Count | | 182 | 64 | 246 |
| | | | % within gender | | 74.0% | 26.0% | 100.0% |

ordinal scale. For example, we may wish to compare the percentage of points where the first serve is in between women's and men's singles matches. In sports performance analysis, the Mann–Whitney U test (like the Wilcoxon test, Kruskal–Wallis H test and the Friedman tests) has typically been used with numerical scale variables. However, it can be used with any dependent variable that can be ranked.

The Mann–Whitney U test is illustrated using the file 'Performances.SAV' to compare women's and men's singles matches in terms of a numerical

Table 8.4(b) Chi square output from SPSS when the file is split on Tournament

**Chi-square tests**

| Tournament | | Value | df | Asymp. Sig. (2-sided) | Exact Sig. (2-sided) | Exact Sig. (1-sided) |
|---|---|---|---|---|---|---|
| Australian Open | Pearson Chi-Square | 1.650[a] | 1 | .199 | | |
| | Continuity Correction[b] | 1.293 | 1 | .256 | | |
| | Likelihood Ratio | 1.656 | 1 | .198 | | |
| | Fisher's Exact Test | | | | .239 | .128 |
| | N of Valid Cases | 241 | | | | |
| French Open | Pearson Chi-Square | 8.340[c] | 1 | .004 | | |
| | Continuity Correction[b] | 7.558 | 1 | .006 | | |
| | Likelihood Ratio | 8.441 | 1 | .004 | | |
| | Fisher's Exact Test | | | | .005 | .003 |
| | N of Valid Cases | 248 | | | | |
| Wimbledon | Pearson Chi-Square | 1.923[d] | 1 | .166 | | |
| | Continuity Correction[b] | 1.553 | 1 | .213 | | |
| | Likelihood Ratio | 1.926 | 1 | .165 | | |
| | Fisher's Exact Test | | | | .206 | .106 |
| | N of Valid Cases | 247 | | | | |
| US Open | Pearson Chi-Square | .432[e] | 1 | .511 | | |
| | Continuity Correction[b] | .262 | 1 | .609 | | |
| | Likelihood Ratio | .432 | 1 | .511 | | |
| | Fisher's Exact Test | | | | .562 | .305 |
| | N of Valid Cases | 246 | | | | |

Notes a. 0 cells (0.0%) have expected count less than 5. The minimum expected count is 30.36.
b. Computed only for a 2x2 table
c. 0 cells (0.0%) have expected count less than 5. The minimum expected count is 36.40.
d. 0 cells (0.0%) have expected count less than 5. The minimum expected count is 35.07.
e. 0 cells (0.0%) have expected count less than 5. The minimum expected count is 31.74.

dependent variable which is the percentage of points where the first serve is in. First, we need the all-important descriptive statistics, which are produced using **Analyse** → **Compare Means** → **Means**, transferring 'Gender' into the Independent Variable area and 'First In' into the Dependent List. When we click on **OK**, SPSS produces the output shown in Table 8.5 which reveals that there is a similar percentage of points where the first serve is in for women's singles (62.0±9.0%) and men's singles (61.3±7.4%). Some choose to show medians and inter-quartile ranges instead of means and standard deviations, especially where dependent variables have skewed distributions.

The small difference of 0.7% between the two means may or may not be significant. We perform a Mann–Whitney U test using **Analyse** → **Nonparametric tests** → **Legacy Dialogs** → **2 Independent Samples**. 'First In' is transferred into the Test Variable List and 'Gender' is transferred into the Grouping variable area. We need to define the groups as 1 and 2 because these are the values we use in the SPSS data sheet to represent female and male players respectively. Tables 8.6(a) and 8.6(b) show the SPSS output for the Mann–Whitney U test. The test has actually found a significant difference between women's and men's singles for the percentage of points where the first serve is in (U = 456373.5, p = 0.034).

This example has pooled data from the four tournaments together. We can analyse the effect of gender on the percentage of points where the first serve was in by logically splitting the file on Tournament so that the gender comparison can be done for all four tournaments separately (**Data** → **Split File**, choose the radio button to compare groups in a single table with groups being based on 'Tournament'). From now on every test we ask for will be applied to the four tournaments separately until we logically un-split the file. We ask for descriptive statistics to compare the means and apply the Mann–Whitney U test identically to how we did it

Table 8.5 Descriptive statistics for independent groups output by SPSS

**Report**

| First In Gender | Mean | N | Std. deviation |
|---|---|---|---|
| Female | 61.950 | 994 | 9.0072 |
| Male | 61.264 | 972 | 7.3801 |
| Total | 61.611 | 1966 | 8.2480 |

Table 8.6(a) SPSS Output for the Mann–Whitney U test: rank

**Ranks**

|  | Gender | N | Mean rank | Sum of ranks |
|---|---|---|---|---|
| First In | Female | 994 | 1010.37 | 1004309.50 |
|  | Male | 972 | 956.02 | 929251.50 |
|  | Total | 1966 |  |  |

Table 8.6(b) SPSS Output for the Mann–Whitney U test: test statistics

**Test statistics[a]**

|  | First In |
|---|---|
| Mann–Whitney U | 456373.500 |
| Wilcoxon W | 929251.500 |
| Z | −2.123 |
| Asymp. Sig. (2-tailed) | .034 |

Note: a. Grouping variable: gender

for the whole file, but this time the output in Tables 8.7, 8.8(a) and 8.8(b) is produced. The only significant difference between men's and women's singles for the percentage of points where the first serve was in was at the US Open (U = 26384.5, p = 0.009).

Table 8.7 Descriptive statistics comparing means when the file is split on Tournament

**Report**

| First In Tournament | Gender | Mean | N | Std. deviation |
|---|---|---|---|---|
| Australian Open | Female | 61.623 | 246 | 8.4066 |
|  | Male | 61.247 | 236 | 7.3840 |
|  | Total | 61.439 | 482 | 7.9164 |
| French Open | Female | 62.124 | 252 | 9.9705 |
|  | Male | 61.259 | 244 | 7.7262 |
|  | Total | 61.698 | 496 | 8.9387 |
| Wimbledon | Female | 63.270 | 250 | 8.5418 |
|  | Male | 63.831 | 244 | 6.2486 |
|  | Total | 63.547 | 494 | 7.4950 |
| US Open | Female | 60.756 | 246 | 8.8771 |
|  | Male | 58.762 | 248 | 7.2322 |
|  | Total | 59.755 | 494 | 8.1464 |

198

**Table 8.8(a)** Mann–Whitney U test results produced by SPSS when the file is logically split on Tournament: ranks

**Ranks**

| Tournament | | Gender | N | Mean rank | Sum of ranks |
|---|---|---|---|---|---|
| Australian Open | First In | Female | 246 | 248.52 | 61136.50 |
| | | Male | 236 | 234.18 | 55266.50 |
| | | Total | 482 | | |
| French Open | First In | Female | 252 | 256.90 | 64740.00 |
| | | Male | 244 | 239.82 | 58516.00 |
| | | Total | 496 | | |
| Wimbledon | First In | Female | 250 | 242.40 | 60600.00 |
| | | Male | 244 | 252.73 | 61665.00 |
| | | Total | 494 | | |
| US Open | First In | Female | 246 | 264.25 | 65004.50 |
| | | Male | 248 | 230.89 | 57260.50 |
| | | Total | 494 | | |

**Table 8.8(b)** Mann–Whitney U test results produced by SPSS when the file is logically split on Tournament: test statistics

**Test statistics[a]**

| Tournament | | First In |
|---|---|---|
| Australian Open | Mann–Whitney U | 27300.500 |
| | Wilcoxon W | 55266.500 |
| | Z | −1.130 |
| | Asymp. Sig. (2-tailed) | .258 |
| French Open | Mann–Whitney U | 28626.000 |
| | Wilcoxon W | 58516.000 |
| | Z | −1.327 |
| | Asymp. Sig. (2-tailed) | .184 |
| Wimbledon | Mann–Whitney U | 29225.000 |
| | Wilcoxon W | 60600.000 |
| | Z | −.804 |
| | Asymp. Sig. (2-tailed) | .422 |
| US Open | Mann–Whitney U | 26384.500 |
| | Wilcoxon W | 57260.500 |
| | Z | −2.597 |
| | Asymp. Sig. (2-tailed) | .009 |

Note: a. Grouping variable: gender

**Exercise 8.3**

Compare the percentage of points won when the first serve is in and when a second serve is required between women's and men's singles matches. Do this for the four Grand Slam tennis tournaments separately.

**Wilcoxon signed-ranks test**

The Wilcoxon singed-ranks test is used to compare two samples drawn from the same cases. The two samples are related samples rather than independent samples. For example, if we wished to compare the percentage of points won between points where the first serve was in and points where a second serve was required, these would be two samples related to the same performances. There are first and second serve points in all tennis matches. The example used to illustrate the Wilcoxon signed-ranks test is a comparison of winning and losing players' performances within matches. These may be different players, but the performances are not independent; a player's performance is clearly influenced by the play of the opponent. Therefore, we consider the winning and losing performances as being different conditions within matches that can be compared. Thus match is the unit of analysis.

This example uses data in the file 'Matches.SAV' and the purpose of the test is to see if there is a difference between the percentage of points where the first serve is in between the winning and losing players within matches. If the file you are using is currently split, then un-split it using **Data → Split** and choose to analyse all cases without creating groups. Unlike the Mann–Whitney U test, we use **Analyse → Descriptive Statistics → Descriptives** to obtain the mean and standard deviation for each sample. This is because the **Compare Means** option is used where we have an independent variable that distinguishes different groups of cases. The two variables we choose are 'W_FirstIn' and 'L_FirstIn'. Table 8.9 shows the SPSS output revealing that the winning players get their first serve in more often, but is this significant?

The Wilcoxon signed-ranks test is done using **Analyse → Nonparametric tests → Legacy dialogs → 2 Related Samples**, transferring 'W_FirstIn' and 'L_FirstIn' into the test pairs area as a pair of related variables. When we click on **OK** the output shown in Tables 8.10(a) and 8.10(b) is produced. Despite the fact that there are 423 of the 982 matches where the losing

**Table 8.9** Descriptive statistics output by SPSS

**Descriptive statistics**

|  | N | Minimum | Maximum | Mean | Std. deviation |
|---|---|---|---|---|---|
| W_FirstIn | 982 | 34.1 | 89.2 | 62.519 | 8.4261 |
| L_FirstIn | 982 | 37.3 | 84.0 | 60.679 | 7.9515 |
| Valid N (listwise) | 982 |  |  |  |  |

player got the first serve in more than the winning player, the result is that the winning player has a significantly greater percentage of service points where the first serve is in than the losing player ($z = -5.1$, $p < 0.001$). Note that the p value of 0.000 to three decimal places is not actually zero. Therefore, this author prefers to express this level of significance as '< 0.001' even though '= 0.000' is technically correct when using three decimal places.

**Table 8.10(a)** SPSS Output for the Wilcoxon signed-ranks test: ranks

**Ranks**

|  |  | N | Mean rank | Sum of ranks |
|---|---|---|---|---|
| L_FirstIn - W_FirstIn | Negative ranks | 555[a] | 512.57 | 284479.00 |
|  | Positive ranks | 423[b] | 459.22 | 194252.00 |
|  | Ties | 4[c] |  |  |
|  | Total | 982 |  |  |

Notes: a. L_FirstIn < W_FirstIn
b. L_FirstIn > W_FirstIn
c. L_FirstIn = W_FirstIn

**Table 8.10(b)** SPSS Output for the Wilcoxon signed-ranks test: test statistics

**Test statistics[a]**

|  | L_FirstIn - W_FirstIn |
|---|---|
| Z | -5.106[b] |
| Asymp. Sig. (2-tailed) | .000 |

Notes: a. Wilcoxon signed-ranks test
b. Based on positive ranks.

The test we have just done used women's and men's singles matches from all four tournaments pooled together. We can compare the percentage of points where the first serve was in between women's and men's singles for the eight different games separately (2 genders × 4 tournaments). This is done by logically splitting the file on gender and tournament (**Data →** **Split File**). The descriptive statistics and Wilcoxon signed-ranks test results when we do this are shown in Tables 8.11, 8.12(a) and 8.12(b). In women's singles, the Australian and French Opens show significant differences between winning and losing players' percentages of points where the first serve was in. In men's singles, the Australian Open and Wimbledon show significant differences between winning and losing players' percentage of points where the first serve was in.

### Exercise 8.4

This may seem obvious but compare the percentage of points won when the first serve is in between winning and losing players for the 2 × 4 (gender × tournament) sets of matches separately. Do the same for the percentage of points won when a second serve is required.

### Kruskal–Wallis H test

The Kruskal–Wallis H test is used to compare three or more independent samples in terms of some dependent variable that is measured on an ordinal or numerical scale. For example, we may have sets of matches played at different tournaments that we wish to compare in terms of the percentage of points where the first serve is in. This example will be illustrated using the 'Performances.SAV' file. We first get the descriptive statistics of interest using **Analyse → Compare Means → Means**, with 'Tournament' being transferred into the Independent variable and 'FirstIn' being transferred into the Dependent List. Table 8.13 shows the means and standard deviations for the four tournaments.

The Kruskal–Wallis H test is done using **Analyse → Nonparametric tests → Legacy Dialogs → K Independent Samples**, transferring 'Tournament' into the Grouping variable area and defining the range of grouping values to be 1 to 4 because these are the values used to represent the four tournaments. 'FirstIn' is transferred into the Test Variable List before we click

Table 8.11 Descriptive statistics for the 4 tournaments for women's and men's singles

**Descriptive statistics**

| Gender | Tournament | | N | Minimum | Maximum | Mean | Std. deviation |
|---|---|---|---|---|---|---|---|
| Female | Australian Open | W_FirstIn | 123 | 37.0 | 79.6 | 63.173 | 8.2628 |
| | | L_FirstIn | 123 | 39.6 | 78.2 | 60.074 | 8.2943 |
| | | Valid N (listwise) | 123 | | | | |
| | French Open | W_FirstIn | 126 | 38.7 | 85.7 | 63.472 | 10.4901 |
| | | L_FirstIn | 126 | 37.3 | 81.5 | 60.778 | 9.2707 |
| | | Valid N (listwise) | 126 | | | | |
| | Wimbledon | W_FirstIn | 125 | 47.8 | 89.0 | 64.226 | 8.5007 |
| | | L_FirstIn | 125 | 37.7 | 83.5 | 62.314 | 8.5086 |
| | | Valid N (listwise) | 125 | | | | |
| | US Open | W_FirstIn | 122 | 34.1 | 89.2 | 61.370 | 9.4171 |
| | | L_FirstIn | 122 | 42.1 | 81.8 | 59.930 | 8.1625 |
| | | Valid N (listwise) | 122 | | | | |
| Male | Australian Open | W_FirstIn | 118 | 44.4 | 88.0 | 62.242 | 7.2904 |
| | | L_FirstIn | 118 | 41.6 | 84.0 | 60.253 | 7.3735 |
| | | Valid N (listwise) | 118 | | | | |
| | French Open | W_FirstIn | 122 | 37.3 | 84.3 | 61.962 | 8.1236 |
| | | L_FirstIn | 122 | 39.3 | 81.4 | 60.555 | 7.2725 |
| | | Valid N (listwise) | 122 | | | | |
| | Wimbledon | W_FirstIn | 122 | 44.0 | 77.6 | 64.551 | 6.2619 |
| | | L_FirstIn | 122 | 48.8 | 80.5 | 63.111 | 6.1770 |
| | | Valid N (listwise) | 122 | | | | |
| | US Open | W_FirstIn | 124 | 42.4 | 76.9 | 59.121 | 7.1292 |
| | | L_FirstIn | 124 | 41.7 | 82.8 | 58.403 | 7.3453 |
| | | Valid N (listwise) | 124 | | | | |

**Table 8.12(a)** Wilcoxon signed-ranks test results for the 4 tournaments for women's and men's singles: ranks

**Ranks**

| Gender | Tournament | | | N | Mean rank | Sum of ranks |
|---|---|---|---|---|---|---|
| Female | Australian Open | L_FirstIn - W_FirstIn | Negative ranks | 69[a] | 70.67 | 4876.50 |
| | | | Positive ranks | 53[b] | 49.56 | 2626.50 |
| | | | Ties | 1[c] | | |
| | | | Total | 123 | | |
| | French Open | L_FirstIn - W_FirstIn | Negative ranks | 70[a] | 70.42 | 4929.50 |
| | | | Positive ranks | 55[b] | 53.55 | 2945.50 |
| | | | Ties | 1[c] | | |
| | | | Total | 126 | | |
| | Wimbledon | L_FirstIn - W_FirstIn | Negative ranks | 74[a] | 62.39 | 4616.50 |
| | | | Positive ranks | 51[b] | 63.89 | 3258.50 |
| | | | Ties | 0[c] | | |
| | | | Total | 125 | | |
| | US Open | L_FirstIn - W_FirstIn | Negative ranks | 60[a] | 66.49 | 3989.50 |
| | | | Positive ranks | 61[b] | 55.60 | 3391.50 |
| | | | Ties | 1[c] | | |
| | | | Total | 122 | | |
| Male | Australian Open | L_FirstIn - W_FirstIn | Negative ranks | 71[a] | 59.48 | 4223.00 |
| | | | Positive ranks | 46[b] | 58.26 | 2680.00 |
| | | | Ties | 1[c] | | |
| | | | Total | 118 | | |
| | French Open | L_FirstIn - W_FirstIn | Negative ranks | 65[a] | 64.21 | 4173.50 |
| | | | Positive ranks | 57[b] | 58.41 | 3329.50 |
| | | | Ties | 0[c] | | |
| | | | Total | 122 | | |

Table 8.12(a) continued

**Ranks**

| Gender | Tournament | | N | Mean rank | Sum of ranks |
|---|---|---|---|---|---|
| | Wimbledon | L_FirstIn - W_FirstIn | | | |
| | | Negative ranks | 74[a] | 61.88 | 4579.00 |
| | | Positive ranks | 48[b] | 60.92 | 2924.00 |
| | | Ties | 0[c] | | |
| | | Total | 122 | | |
| | US Open | L_FirstIn - W_FirstIn | | | |
| | | Negative ranks | 72[a] | 61.47 | 4425.50 |
| | | Positive ranks | 52[b] | 63.93 | 3324.50 |
| | | Ties | 0[c] | | |
| | | Total | 124 | | |

Notes: a. L_FirstIn < W_FirstIn
b. L_FirstIn > W_FirstIn
c. L_FirstIn = W_FirstIn

**Table 8.12(b)** Wilcoxon signed-ranks test results for the 4 tournaments for women's and men's singles: statistics

**Test statistics[a]**

| Gender | Tournament | | L_FirstIn - W_FirstIn |
|--------|-----------|---|----------------------|
| Female | Australian Open | Z | −2.874[b] |
| | | Asymp. Sig. (2-tailed) | .004 |
| | French Open | Z | −2.444[b] |
| | | Asymp. Sig. (2-tailed) | .015 |
| | Wimbledon | Z | −1.673[b] |
| | | Asymp. Sig. (2-tailed) | .094 |
| | US Open | Z | −.773[b] |
| | | Asymp. Sig. (2-tailed) | .439 |
| Male | Australian Open | Z | −2.098[b] |
| | | Asymp. Sig. (2-tailed) | .036 |
| | French Open | Z | −1.078[b] |
| | | Asymp. Sig. (2-tailed) | .281 |
| | Wimbledon | Z | −2.114[b] |
| | | Asymp. Sig. (2-tailed) | .034 |
| | US Open | Z | −1.373[b] |
| | | Asymp. Sig. (2-tailed) | .170 |

Notes: a. Wilcoxon signed-ranks test
b. Based on positive ranks

**Table 8.13** Descriptive statistics for the four different tournaments

**Report**

First In

| Tournament | Mean | N | Std. deviation |
|-----------|------|---|----------------|
| Australian Open | 61.439 | 482 | 7.9164 |
| French Open | 61.698 | 496 | 8.9387 |
| Wimbledon | 63.547 | 494 | 7.4950 |
| US Open | 59.755 | 494 | 8.1464 |
| Total | 61.611 | 1966 | 8.2480 |

on OK obtaining the SPSS output shown in Tables 8.14(a) and 8.14(b). There is a significant difference between the four tournaments ($H_3 = 59.8$, $p < 0.001$). Note that where there are at least five cases in each sample being compared, the H statistic approximates to the chi square distribution. Some authors report this as $\chi^2$ while others use H.

**Table 8.14(a)** SPSS output for the Kruskal–Wallis H test: ranks

**Ranks**

| Tournament | | N | Mean rank |
|---|---|---|---|
| First In | Australian Open | 482 | 974.57 |
| | French Open | 496 | 989.39 |
| | Wimbledon | 494 | 1124.31 |
| | US Open | 494 | 845.49 |
| | Total | 1966 | |

**Table 8.14(b)** SPSS output for the Kruskal–Wallis H test: test statistics

**Test Statistics[a,b]**

| | First In |
|---|---|
| Chi-Square | 59.765 |
| Df | 3 |
| Asymp. Sig. | .000 |

Notes: a. Kruskal–Wallis test
b. Grouping variable: Tournament

There is a significant difference between the tournaments, but the Kruskal–Wallis H test does not tell us which pairs of tournaments are significantly different. Therefore, we should use follow up Mann–Whitney U tests to compare the different pairs of tournaments. Remember, the four tournaments are considered to be independent samples and, therefore, any pairs of tournaments would consist of two independent samples. This means the Mann–Whitney U test should be used for follow-up pairwise comparisons rather than the Wilcoxon signed-ranks test. There are four tournaments and so there are six pairs of tournaments. A Bonferroni adjustment can be applied to the p value required to achieve a significant difference in the post hoc tests to avoid Type I Error inflation. The easiest way to set this is to divide the usual threshold p value (say 0.05) by the number of pairwise tests to be done (in this case 6). Therefore, only p values less than 0.008 from the follow-up Mann–Whitney U tests will be considered significant. When these tests are done, all pairs of tournaments are significantly different (p < 0.001) except the Australia and French Opens (p = 0.687).

The comparison of tournaments that we have just done pooled women's and men's singles matches together. When the file is logically split on gender and the analysis is repeated, we obtain the descriptive statistics in Table 8.15 and the Kruskal–Wallis H test results shown in Tables 8.16(a) and 8.16(b) respectively. As we can see, tournament has a significant influence on the percentage of points where the first serve was in for both women's ($H_3 = 11.0$, $p = 0.012$) and men's singles ($H_3 = 65.3$, $p < 0.001$). Post hoc Mann–Whitney U tests for women's singles revealed that only Wimbledon and US Open were significantly different ($p < 0.001$); the others had p values ranging from 0.054 to 0.570 and would not be significant even if we were not using a Bonferroni adjustment. The post hoc Mann–Whitney U tests for men's singles found no significant difference between the Australia and French Open ($p = 0.902$), but all other pairs of tournaments were significantly different ($p < 0.001$).

## Exercise 8.5

Compare the percentage of points that were won when the first serve was in between the four tournaments for women's and men's singles separately. Do follow-up pairwise comparisons between pairs of tournaments if tournament has a significant effect. Repeat this analysis for the percentage of points won when a second serve is required.

Table 8.15 Tournament means and standard deviations for women's and men's singles

**Report**

| First In Gender | Tournament | Mean | N | Std. deviation |
|---|---|---|---|---|
| Female | Australian Open | 61.623 | 246 | 8.4066 |
| | French Open | 62.124 | 252 | 9.9705 |
| | Wimbledon | 63.270 | 250 | 8.5418 |
| | US Open | 60.756 | 246 | 8.8771 |
| | Total | 61.950 | 994 | 9.0072 |
| Male | Australian Open | 61.247 | 236 | 7.3840 |
| | French Open | 61.259 | 244 | 7.7262 |
| | Wimbledon | 63.831 | 244 | 6.2486 |
| | US Open | 58.762 | 248 | 7.2322 |
| | Total | 61.264 | 972 | 7.3801 |

208

**Table 8.16(a)** Kruskal–Wallis H test results for women's and men's singles separately: ranks

**Ranks**

| Gender | | Tournament | N | Mean rank |
|--------|--|-----------|---|-----------|
| Female | First In | Australian Open | 246 | 491.90 |
| | | French Open | 252 | 506.00 |
| | | Wimbledon | 250 | 537.67 |
| | | US Open | 246 | 453.57 |
| | | Total | 994 | |
| Male | First In | Australian Open | 236 | 480.83 |
| | | French Open | 244 | 483.77 |
| | | Wimbledon | 244 | 593.48 |
| | | US Open | 248 | 389.32 |
| | | Total | 972 | |

**Table 8.16(b)** Kruskal–Wallis H test results for women's and men's singles separately: test statistics

**Test statistics**[a,b]

| Gender | | | First In |
|--------|--|--|----------|
| Female | Chi-Square | | 10.971 |
| | df | | 3 |
| | Asymp. Sig. | | .012 |
| Male | Chi-Square | | 65.271 |
| | df | | 3 |
| | Asymp. Sig. | | .000 |

Notes: a. Kruskal–Wallis test
     b. Grouping variable: Tournament

## Freidman test

The Friedman test is used to compare three or more samples related to the same cases. For example we may wish to compare passing statistics for a group of basketball players between the four quarters of a game. The samples are typically repeated measurements of some conceptual dependent variable. The repeated measures could be made at different times or under different conditions. Despite using tournament effect on the percentage of points where the first serve is in as an example of the Kruskal–Wallis H test, we will also use this as an example of the

Friedman test. The difference is that the Friedman test needs data from the four different tournaments for the same set of players. This also makes a point that there are alternative research designs, units of analysis and statistical tests that can be applied to the same research question. This example uses data in the file 'Tournament comparison.SAV' where we have data from at least 3 matches per tournament for the 15 players included in the file. The 'A_', 'F_', 'W_' and 'U_' prefixes are used to signify the different tournaments (Australian Open, French Open, Wimbledon and US Open respectively).

First the means and standard deviations for the percentage of points where the players played the first serve in at the four tournaments are obtained using **Analyse → Descriptive Statistics → Descriptives** entering 'A_FirstIn', 'F_FirstIn', 'W_FirstIn' and 'U_FirstIn' into the Test Variable List. This gives the output shown in Table 8.17.

The Friedman test is done using **Analyse → Nonparametric tests → Legacy Dialogs → K Related Samples** entering 'A_FirstIn', 'F_FirstIn', 'W_FirstIn' and 'U_FirstIn' into the Test Variables. This produces the results shown in Tables 8.18(a) and 8.18(b), revealing that the players did play their first serves in on a significantly different percentage of points between the four tournaments ($\chi^2_3 = 12.4$, p = 0.006).

Because we have found a significant difference between the tournaments, we use follow-up Wilcoxon signed-ranks tests to compare the six pairs of tournaments (**Analyse → Nonparametric tests → Legacy Dialogs → 2 Related Samples**). The four tournaments are four different conditions experienced by all 15 players. Therefore, each pair of tournaments involves two conditions to be compared within the sample of players. We can enter all six pairs of tournaments into a single popup when doing

Table 8.17 Descriptive statistics for the percentage of points where the first serve was in at the four tournaments

**Descriptive statistics**

|  | N | Minimum | Maximum | Mean | Std. deviation |
|---|---|---|---|---|---|
| A_First In | 15 | 57.8 | 69.8 | 62.607 | 3.5391 |
| F_First In | 15 | 48.2 | 74.7 | 64.142 | 6.4971 |
| W_First In | 15 | 60.1 | 72.9 | 66.502 | 3.1344 |
| U_First In | 15 | 49.1 | 67.2 | 60.921 | 5.5516 |
| Valid N (listwise) | 15 |  |  |  |  |

**Table 8.18(a)** Friedman test results from SPSS: ranks

**Ranks**

|  | Mean rank |
|---|---|
| A_First In | 2.13 |
| F_First In | 2.73 |
| W_First In | 3.33 |
| U_First In | 1.80 |

**Table 8.18(b)** Friedman test results from SPSS: test statistics

**Test statistics[a]**

|  |  |
|---|---|
| N | 15 |
| Chi-Square | 12.360 |
| Df | 3 |
| Asymp. Sig. | .006 |

Note: a. Friedman Test

these follow-up Wilcoxon signed-ranks tests; this is better than what we had to do with the Mann-Whitney U tests that followed the Kruskal Wallis H test. The results of these Wilcoxon tests are shown in Tables 8.19(a) and 8.19(b). Using a Bonferroni adjustment ($p < 0.008$), the percentage of points where the first serve is in was significantly greater at Wimbledon than at the Australian and US Open tournaments.

This analysis pooled the female and male players into a single sample. We may wish to compare the tournaments within the sample of female and male players separately by splitting the file on gender (**Data → Split File**). Table 8.20 shows the SPSS output for the descriptive statistics and Tables 8.21(a) and 8.21(b) show the output for the Friedman tests for the female and male players. There was a significant difference for the percentage of points where the first serve was in between the tournaments for the male players ($\chi^2_3 = 10.2$, $p = 0.019$) but not the female players ($\chi^2_3 = 4.2$, $p = 0.241$). However, the pairwise Wilcoxon signed-ranks comparisons for men did not find significant differences between any pair of tournaments ($p > 0.011$); remember we are using a Bonferroni adjustment requiring p values of less than 0.008 to indicate a significant difference between pairs of tournaments.

**Table 8.19(a)** SPSS output for follow-up Wilcoxon signed-ranks tests comparing pairs of tournaments: ranks

**Ranks**

| | | N | Mean rank | Sum of ranks |
|---|---|---|---|---|
| F_First In - A_First In | Negative ranks | 6[a] | 6.67 | 40.00 |
| | Positive ranks | 9[b] | 8.89 | 80.00 |
| | Ties | 0[c] | | |
| | Total | 15 | | |
| W_First In - A_First In | Negative ranks | 2[d] | 2.50 | 5.00 |
| | Positive ranks | 13[e] | 8.85 | 115.00 |
| | Ties | 0[f] | | |
| | Total | 15 | | |
| U_First In - A_First In | Negative ranks | 9[g] | 8.67 | 78.00 |
| | Positive ranks | 6[h] | 7.00 | 42.00 |
| | Ties | 0[i] | | |
| | Total | 15 | | |
| W_First In - F_First In | Negative ranks | 6[j] | 6.00 | 36.00 |
| | Positive ranks | 9[k] | 9.33 | 84.00 |
| | Ties | 0[l] | | |
| | Total | 15 | | |
| U_First In - F_First In | Negative ranks | 11[m] | 8.73 | 96.00 |
| | Positive ranks | 4[n] | 6.00 | 24.00 |
| | Ties | 0[o] | | |
| | Total | 15 | | |
| U_First In - W_First In | Negative ranks | 13[p] | 8.92 | 116.00 |
| | Positive ranks | 2[q] | 2.00 | 4.00 |
| | Ties | 0[r] | | |
| | Total | 15 | | |

Notes: a. F_First In < A_First In
b. F_First In > A_First In
c. F_First In = A_First In
d. W_First In < A_First In
e. W_First In > A_First In
f. W_First In = A_First In
g. U_First In < A_First In
h. U_First In > A_First In
i. U_First In = A_First In
j. W_First In < F_First In
k. W_First In > F_First In
l. W_First In = F_First In
m. U_First In < F_First In
n. U_First In > F_First In
o. U_First In = F_First In
p. U_First In < W_First In
q. U_First In > W_First In
r. U_First In = W_First In

**Table 8.19(b)** SPSS output for follow-up Wilcoxon signed-ranks tests comparing pairs of tournaments: test statistics

**Test statistics[a]**

| | F_First In – A_First In | W_First In – A_First In | U_First In – A_First In | W_First In – F_First In | U_First In – F_First In | U_First In – W_First In |
|---|---|---|---|---|---|---|
| Z | −1.136[b] | −3.124[b] | −1.022[c] | −1.363[b] | −2.045[c] | −3.181[c] |
| Asymp. Sig. (2-tailed) | .256 | .002 | .307 | .173 | .041 | .001 |

Notes: a. Wilcoxon signed-ranks test
b. Based on negative ranks.
c. Based on positive ranks.

**Table 8.20** Descriptive statistics for a set of female and male players at different tournaments

**Descriptive statistics**

| Gender | | N | Minimum | Maximum | Mean | Std. deviation |
|---|---|---|---|---|---|---|
| Female | A_First In | 6 | 60.4 | 69.8 | 65.098 | 3.3503 |
| | F_First In | 6 | 48.2 | 74.7 | 65.083 | 9.5540 |
| | W_First In | 6 | 64.9 | 72.9 | 67.286 | 3.2993 |
| | U_First In | 6 | 49.1 | 67.1 | 61.869 | 6.6412 |
| | Valid N (listwise) | 6 | | | | |
| Male | A_First In | 9 | 57.8 | 65.3 | 60.945 | 2.6727 |
| | F_First In | 9 | 58.6 | 71.4 | 63.515 | 3.9644 |
| | W_First In | 9 | 60.1 | 69.3 | 65.980 | 3.1019 |
| | U_First In | 9 | 51.6 | 67.2 | 60.289 | 5.0247 |
| | Valid N (listwise) | 9 | | | | |

**Table 8.21(a)** Friedman test results for female and male players separately: ranks

**Ranks**

| Gender | | Mean rank |
|---|---|---|
| Female | A_First In | 2.50 |
| | F_First In | 2.33 |
| | W_First In | 3.33 |
| | U_First In | 1.83 |
| Male | A_First In | 1.89 |
| | F_First In | 3.00 |
| | W_First In | 3.33 |
| | U_First In | 1.78 |

**Table 8.21(b)** Friedman test results for female and male players separately: test statistics

**Test statistics[a]**

| | | |
|---|---|---|
| Female | N | 6 |
| | Chi-Square | 4.200 |
| | Df | 3 |
| | Asymp. Sig. | .241 |
| Male | N | 9 |
| | Chi-Square | 9.933 |
| | Df | 3 |
| | Asymp. Sig. | .019 |

Note: a. Friedman Test

## Exercise 8.6

Compare the percentage of points won when the first serve is in between the four tournaments for the female players and male players separately in the file 'Tournament comparison'. Where there is a significant tournament effect, use appropriate tests to compare each pair of tournaments. Repeat the analysis for the percentage of points won when a second serve is required.

## Spearman's rho

Spearman's $\rho$ is a rank-based correlation technique that is sometimes used with sports performance data to evaluate the strength and direction of relationships between variables. For example, we might want to look at the relationship between the percentage of points won when the first serve is in and the percentage of points won when a second serve is required. One might expect these to be positively related because once a rally develops, both types of point depend on the ability to play winners and avoid errors. We will use this as an example of Spearman's $\rho$ applying it to the data in the 'Performances.SAV' file. The data can initially be explored using a scatter plot by using the menu **Graphs** → **Chart Builder**. A message pops up about measurement levels and scales being correct before using chart builder with any variables; the data in the 'Performances.SAV' file are fine. Click on **OK**.

214

Choose 'Scatter/Dot' in the 'Choose from area'. A set of tiles will appear. We choose the one with different colours of dots; this will ensure that women's and men's data are shown in different colours. Drag the second tile on the top row of tiles into the preview area. A template for our scatter plot appears in the preview area with areas to drag variables into. Drag 'Won1' into x-axis label, 'Won2' into y-axis label and 'Gender' into Set Colour. The chart shown in Figure 8.6 is produced.

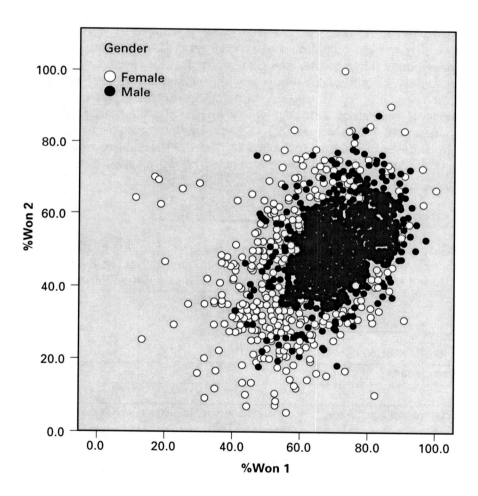

Figure 8.6 Scatter plot produced by SPSS

The relationship between the two variables looks positive but weak. The male data seems more consistent than women's data. Correlation coefficients are produced using **Analyse** → **Correlate** → **Bivariate**, removing the tick from Pearson and putting a tick in Spearman. Drag 'Won1' and 'Won2' to the variables area. Then click on **OK** and the output shown in Table 8.22 appears. An absolute rank correlation of under 0.2 represents no correlation between the two variables while a rank correlation of over 0.7 represents a strong relationship between the variables.

There is a positive relationship ($\rho$ = +.436) but any strength in the correlation may be explained by there being two overlapping clusters of data for women's and men's singles with the men winning a greater percentage of points on both first and second serve than women. Similarly, players may win a greater percentage of points on serve at one tournament than the others. The gender and tournament factors can be removed from correlation by determining correlations for the 2 genders × 4 tournaments separately. This requires us to split the file both gender and tournament. When we do this and ask for the correlations again, we obtain the output shown in Table 8.23. Three of the eight correlations are actually higher than the +0.436 produced for the whole data set.

**Exercise 8.7**

We speculate that the more likely a serve is to be in, the less likely it is that the point will be won if the serve is in. Serves that are always in are soft and the receiving player can take advantage of this. Serves that are

Table 8.22 SPSS output for Spearman's $\rho$

**Correlations**

| | | | %Won 1 | %Won 2 |
|---|---|---|---|---|
| Spearman's $\rho$ | %Won 1 | Correlation coefficient | 1.000 | .436** |
| | | Sig. (2-tailed) | . | .000 |
| | | N | 1966 | 1966 |
| | %Won 2 | Correlation coefficient | .436** | 1.000 |
| | | Sig. (2-tailed) | .000 | . |
| | | N | 1966 | 1966 |

Note: **. Correlation is significant at the 0.01 level (2-tailed).

Table 8.23 SPSS output for Spearman's ρ for each combination of gender and tournament

**Correlations**

| Gender | Tournament | | | | %Won 1 | %Won 2 |
|---|---|---|---|---|---|---|
| Female | Australian Open | Spearman's ρ | %Won 1 | Correlation coefficient | 1.000 | .335** |
| | | | | Sig. (2-tailed) | . | .000 |
| | | | | N | 246 | 246 |
| | | | %Won 2 | Correlation coefficient | .335** | 1.000 |
| | | | | Sig. (2-tailed) | .000 | . |
| | | | | N | 246 | 246 |
| | French Open | Spearman's ρ | %Won 1 | Correlation coefficient | 1.000 | .255** |
| | | | | Sig. (2-tailed) | . | .000 |
| | | | | N | 252 | 252 |
| | | | %Won 2 | Correlation coefficient | .255** | 1.000 |
| | | | | Sig. (2-tailed) | .000 | . |
| | | | | N | 252 | 252 |
| | Wimbledon | Spearman's ρ | %Won 1 | Correlation coefficient | 1.000 | .377** |
| | | | | Sig. (2-tailed) | . | .000 |
| | | | | N | 250 | 250 |
| | | | %Won 2 | Correlation coefficient | .377** | 1.000 |
| | | | | Sig. (2-tailed) | .000 | . |
| | | | | N | 250 | 250 |
| | US Open | Spearman's ρ | %Won 1 | Correlation coefficient | 1.000 | .449** |
| | | | | Sig. (2-tailed) | . | .000 |
| | | | | N | 246 | 246 |
| | | | %Won 2 | Correlation coefficient | .449** | 1.000 |
| | | | | Sig. (2-tailed) | .000 | . |
| | | | | N | 246 | 246 |

Table 8.23 continued

| Gender | Tournament | | | | %Won 1 | %Won 2 |
|---|---|---|---|---|---|---|
| Male | Australian Open | Spearman's ρ | %Won 1 | Correlation coefficient | 1.000 | .445** |
| | | | | Sig. (2-tailed) | . | .000 |
| | | | | N | 236 | 236 |
| | | | %Won 2 | Correlation coefficient | .445** | 1.000 |
| | | | | Sig. (2-tailed) | .000 | . |
| | | | | N | 236 | 236 |
| | French Open | Spearman's ρ | %Won 1 | Correlation coefficient | 1.000 | .449** |
| | | | | Sig. (2-tailed) | . | .000 |
| | | | | N | 244 | 244 |
| | | | %Won 2 | Correlation coefficient | .449** | 1.000 |
| | | | | Sig. (2-tailed) | .000 | . |
| | | | | N | 244 | 244 |
| | Wimbledon | Spearman's ρ | %Won 1 | Correlation coefficient | 1.000 | .342** |
| | | | | Sig. (2-tailed) | . | .000 |
| | | | | N | 244 | 244 |
| | | | %Won 2 | Correlation coefficient | .342** | 1.000 |
| | | | | Sig. (2-tailed) | .000 | . |
| | | | | N | 244 | 244 |
| | US Open | Spearman's ρ | %Won 1 | Correlation coefficient | 1.000 | .405** |
| | | | | Sig. (2-tailed) | . | .000 |
| | | | | N | 248 | 248 |
| | | | %Won 2 | Correlation coefficient | .405** | 1.000 |
| | | | | Sig. (2-tailed) | .000 | . |
| | | | | N | 248 | 248 |

Note: **. Correlation is significant at the 0.01 level (2-tailed)

rarely in are played at speed, aiming close to the lines and are more difficult to return in court. This suggests a relationship between the percentage of points where the first serve is in and the percentage of points won when the first serve is in should be negatively correlated. Produce a scatter plot with 'FirstIn' on the x-axis and 'Won1' on the Y axis. Use different colours of dots for women's and men's data. Now do 2 ×4 (gender × tournament) Spearman's ρ correlations between 'FirstIn' and 'Won1'.

## SUMMARY

This chapter intentionally commenced by describing the process of preparing data for analysis within a statistics package. This is an important step that typically takes longer than the statistical analysis itself. The statistical procedures to be used depend on the units of analysis, whether samples are independent or related, whether we are testing relationships or differences and the design of the study. Some use chi square analysing data at an event level. This can lead to significant results from very few performances and should be avoided. However, chi square can be used legitimately with categorical variables relating to whole performances (for example whether a match was an upset or not). Numerical variables in sports performance analysis are typically compared between samples using non-parametric tests. This is because sports performance data regularly violate the assumptions of parametric procedures. The tests used are the Mann–Whitney U test, Wilcoxon signed-ranks test, Kruskal–Wallis H test and Friedman test. Similarly, when correlations are assessed between sports performance variables, ranked correlations such as Spearman's ρ are used. There are different ways of answering the same research question. For example, in this chapter we showed two different analyses of tournament effect on performance variables. In one example, the Kruskal–Wallis H test was used to compare independent sets of matches from different tournaments. In the other example, a Friedman test considered the tournaments to be conditions experienced by a set of players who had competed at three or more matches in all four tournaments. When analysing data, inferential procedures are important, but researchers should not neglect the all-important descriptive statistics.

# CHAPTER 9

## RELIABILITY

### INTRODUCTION

Reliability is dealt with in different ways by the different disciplines within sports science (O'Donoghue, 2012: 338–41). A physiologist might use a test-retest study to evaluate the reliability of some test. This involves the same set of participants performing the same test on two or more occasions with reliability being based on the correlation or consistency between the different sets of test measures. Sports performance analysts would not use such an approach because sports performance is neither controlled nor stable in the way that fitness tests and anthropometric measures are. There is a great deal of match-to-match variability that results from many factors, most notably the quality of opposition. Therefore, sports performance analysts tend to use independent observations of the same performance(s) within reliability studies. This is referred to as inter-rater reliability.

In sports psychology, questionnaire instruments are used to produce numerical scores for constructs. Some of these instruments have several dimensions that are also measured by some numerical score derived from the responses to questions. The reliability of such constructs can be evaluated be measuring internal consistency using statistics such as Cronbach's alpha (O'Donoghue, 2012: 364–5). This correlates dimension scores for a set of respondents with high correlations indicating that the different dimensions of the construct are related and hence the overall construct is based on dimensions that are consistent. Sports performance analysts would not use such an approach because they have a different view of what reliability is and the nature of sports performance differs to that of constructs used in sports psychology. Sports performance analysts would not use a correlation between completely different performances measures (such as the percentage of passes successfully completed and the percentage of tackles that are successfully made) because they are different variables. The sports performance analyst wishes to know if each of these variables has been recorded reliably. A performance profile in sports performance includes different aspects of sports performance that are not always expected to be related. For example, a performance profile for a tennis performance might consist of variables representing serving performance, receiving, forehand performance, backhand performance, baseline performance, net performance and break points performance. One player might be relatively strong when serving and relatively weak when receiving compared to another player. A player might be relatively strong at the baseline but relatively weak at the net compared to another player. In team games, some players have positional roles that necessitate specific strengths that are not required by players in other positional roles. For these reasons we cannot expect the variables that comprise a performance profile to be correlated in the way that the dimensions of a construct used in sports psychology are.

A further type of reliability used in sports science is parallel forms reliability, where a measure is correlated with some gold standard measure. Many in performance analysis as well as sports science, in general, would regard such a study as a validation study rather than a reliability study. However, in sports performance analysis, there have been such validation studies done where it is not feasible to conduct a reliability study. For example, it is not practical or economic to install two copies of the Prozone3 player tracking system (Prozone, Sports Ltd, Leeds, UK) at a stadium. Therefore, Di Salvo et al. (2006) validated measures made by Prozone3 against those made by electronic timing gates and O'Donoghue and Robinson (2009) validated Prozone3 data against data gathered by a manual observation process that had good reliability. The idea here is that if a method can be validated against some other reliable method then a case can be made through inductive reasoning that the method must be sufficiently reliable. Therefore, the current chapter will discuss some aspects of conducting validation studies as well as reliability studies in sports performance analysis.

The equations of various statistical tests are covered in other books. For example, the use of percentage error, chi square and correlation techniques are described by Hughes et al. (2004). O'Donoghue (2010: 161–77) has described the use of kappa, mean absolute error and 95 per cent limits of agreement within reliability studies of performance analysis systems. The use of percentage error, kappa and mean absolute error is also described in Chapter 9 of O'Donoghue's (2015) textbook. Therefore, the main purpose of the current chapter is to cover specific processing tasks that are required to produce data in the form where the reliability equations can be applied. The chapter is made up of three broad sections. The first section is specifically about pre-processing data from commercial video analysis packages, such as Sportscode and Focus X2, for the purpose of reliability assessment. The final step of producing the appropriate reliability statistics is also covered in this section. The second section describes how the reliability of special purpose systems, such as Prozone's systems and Opta, has been investigated. The third section considers how to establish the reliability of sports performance data that are available on official tournament websites.

## GENERIC MATCH ANALYSIS SYSTEMS

### Frequency tables

When we use commercial video analysis packages, such as Sportscode, Darfish, Nacsport or Focus X2, we have standard means of entering data, analysing data and producing statistical and video sequence output. This allows the packages to be used in consistent ways with a familiar interface no matter what type of specific sport system is implemented. The packages do not usually provide facilities for reliability assessment, although some like Observer Pro have done. The reason for some packages not covering reliability is that they cannot be all things to all people and provide every type of reliability analysis that might be required for individual systems implemented on the packages. However, the packages' normal outputs do provide the relevant data to allow analysts to conduct whatever type of reliability study they need to with the reliability statistics being calculated in other packages such as Microsoft Excel. The first type of output that can be used in a reliability study is frequency data. Where a system is used during two independent observations of the same performance, two sets of frequency data can be produced and compared. In Focus X2, a Results Grid allows two categories of the system's Category Set to be cross-tabulated with frequencies being displayed. The Results Grid can then be exported for use in a reliability study outside the package itself. Results Grids for different observations can then be compared using percentage error for example. Similarly, Sportscode provides a Matrix of events by value labels, which can be exported as an excel file. Data from Excel files containing matrices for different observations of the same performance can be combined to allow comparison using percentage error. Dartfish and Nacsport also provide the ability to export event frequency data for use in reliability studies.

## Event lists

The frequency data produced in Results Grids (Focus X2) and Matrices (SportsCode and Nacsport) can be used to determine percentage error statistics for reliability. However, kappa cannot be produced from total frequencies as disagreements in values between corresponding event records are not shown. Percentage error has the advantage of being applied to system outputs, which we may wish to certify for reliability. The disadvantage of percentage error is that corresponding frequencies might conceal disagreements that are cancelled out by other disagreements. For example, on one occasion one observer might record an event as a pass and the other might record it as a shot, but on a subsequent occasion they might do this the other way round. This could result in the observers recording the same total frequency for passes and recording the same total frequency for shots despite there being two disagreements in event type. In order to identify such disagreements, we need to use a cross-tabulation of event types (or some other variable) recorded during two independent observations of a performance. This requires the two Event Lists and the use of pivot tables.

Event Lists can be exported from all of the commercial video analysis packages. In Focus X2, the Event List contains a row for each event as well as a column for event time and each category in the given system's Category Set. This has a distinct advantage that columns, containing the values recorded for given categories, correspond to given performance variables. For example, in a tennis system we may have categories for serving player, point type, whether the point was on first or second serve, whether it was served to the Deuce or Advantage court and the outcome of the point. There will be a column for each of these variables in an exported Event List. Values will be placed in the correct column irrespective of whether data are entered in the same category order from one event to another or not.

An Event List (edit list) exported from SportsCode will have three columns for start time, end time and event type of recorded event instances. The fourth column shows which occurrence of the given event type the particular row represents (the 1st, 2nd, 3rd, 4th, ... Nth ...). The fifth column shows the number of value labels recorded for the given instance. However, the value labels that were used within events are recorded in the order in which they were entered. Some events may have more value labels than others, meaning that there are differing row lengths. For example, we may have event types for the different combinations of server and court served to with service, point type and outcome being value labels. If we have a value label '2nd serve' to distinguish between points where a second serve is required, then some point instances will include this label and others will not. This will cause varying record lengths within our edit list. A further issue is that if '2nd serve' is recorded before the point type and outcome, then point type values and outcome values will appear in different columns in first serve points than they do in second serve points. This is illustrated in Figure 9.1.

In a situation like this we can use the number of value labels recorded in Column E to help us produce additional columns where each column does represent a specific variable. In this example we will create new

| | D | E | | | F | G | H | I |
|---|---|---|---|---|---|---|---|---|
| 1 | Start time | End time | Event type | Instance | Label count | Labels | | |
| 2 | 00:0:10:0 | 00:0:15:0 | Plr A Deuce | 1 | 2 | Ace | Won | |
| 3 | 00:0:33:96 | 00:1:0:39 | Plr A Adv | 1 | 3 | 2nd serve | Baseline | Won |
| 4 | 00:1:20:62 | 00:1:33:39 | Plr A Deuce | 2 | 3 | 2nd serve | D Fault | Lost |
| 5 | 00:1:52:75 | 00:2:5:20 | Plr A Adv | 2 | 2 | Baseline | Won | |
| 6 | 00:2:25:71 | 00:2:33:6 | Plr A Deuce | 3 | 2 | Net | Lost | |
| 7 | 00:2:53:37 | 00:3:10:91 | Plr A Adv | 3 | 2 | Baseline | Won | |
| 8 | 00:4:17:39 | 00:4:35:71 | Plr B Deuce | 1 | 2 | Baseline | Won | |
| 9 | 00:4:55:3 | 00:5:21:57 | Plr B Adv | 1 | 3 | 2nd serve | Baseline | Won |
| 10 | 00:5:41:1 | 00:5:45:44 | Plr B Deuce | 2 | 2 | Ace | Won | |
| 11 | 00:6:4:56 | 00:6:14:56 | Plr B Adv | 2 | 2 | Net | Won | |
| 12 | 00:6:55:75 | 00:7:21:7 | Plr A Deuce | 4 | 3 | 2nd serve | Baseline | Lost |
| 13 | 00:7:42:51 | 00:7:54:94 | Plr A Adv | 4 | 2 | Net | Lost | |
| 14 | 00:8:14:55 | 00:8:33:64 | Plr A Deuce | 5 | 2 | Baseline | Won | |
| 15 | 00:8:52:73 | 00:9:9:15 | Plr A Adv | 5 | 3 | 2nd serve | D Fault | Lost |
| 16 | 00:9:27:60 | 00:10:13:36 | Plr A Deuce | 6 | 3 | 2nd serve | Baseline | Won |
| 17 | 00:10:35:32 | 00:10:43:32 | Plr A Adv | 6 | 2 | Baseline | Lost | |

Figure 9.1 An edit list for tennis exported from SportsCode

224

columns for service (Column J), point type (Column K) and outcome (Column L). This can be done as follows:

Cell J2: = IF(E2 = 2, "1st serve", "2nd serve")
Cell K2: = IF(E2 = 2, F2, G2)
Cell L2: = IF(E2 = 2, G2, H2)

The functions in these three cells can then be copied and pasted into the remaining rows giving the three variables. Note that this approach works for the current example where the user has entered the value labels for 2nd service (if required), point type and outcome in a consistent order within the point instances.

More complex systems can give rise to greater difficulty in converting an Edit List into a form suitable for processing with pivot tables within a reliability study. We need to consider such issues when designing systems. An important aspect of the system is that it is usable and reflects the operator's mental model of events being entered. This should not be compromised in order to ease the processing of the reliability study. It is essential that the reliability study is carried out using observations conducted in the way they would be when the system is used in practice. The operator activity during data collection is part of the system and not separate to it. If we change this (by enforcing a specific ordering in which labels are entered) just for the reliability study, then the reliability study is not being applied to the exact system that will be used in practice.

Once the columns for specific variables have been created in the Edit Lists from each independent observation, the observations can be combined with pivot tables used to cross-tabulate the two observer's data for each variable in turn. This then allows the kappa statistic to be determined for each variable in as described by O'Donoghue (2012: 348).

## Mismatching event lists

The previously used example of tennis points is one where independent observers, typically at least, agree on the number of events (tennis points) that have occurred. However, there are many types of analysis where independent observers rarely agree on the number of events performed. Two examples that are discussed in this chapter are

Prozone's MatchViewer system and the OPTA Sportsdata statistics used in soccer.

Liu *et al.* (2013) did an inter-operator agreement study for OPTA Sportsdata. The system actually uses operator pairs with separate operators coding the events performed by each team in a match. Liu *et al.*'s study compared the data recorded by independent operator pairs for a single soccer match. There were 1547 events that were recorded by both pairs of observers with an additional 15 events recorded by the first pair but not the second and an additional 38 events recorded by the second pair but not the first. This means that we cannot simply take the two raw event lists and use them to create a series of pivot tables (one pivot table for each variable). We need to match the events up. Liu *et al.* (2013) did this and calculated kappa values including situations where events were recorded by single observer pairs as well as those recorded by both. This meant that there were occasions where events recorded by one observer pair disagreed with 'no event recorded' by the other. However, there was no figure recorded for agreements for 'no event recorded'. This makes this version of the kappa statistic quite a harsh reliability statistic, but this does give greater confidence in high kappa values when they are produced. The actual calculation of kappa, once we have cross-tabulated event frequencies, is the same as if we did not have the additional 'no event recorded' value. Therefore, the remainder of this section will discuss the event matching process.

Table 9.1 is an example of a match section where mismatches have been identified. For example, there are 3 events at 591.2s to 593.8s that were identified in Observation 2 but not in Observation 1. Similarly, there was an event at 601.4s that was identified in Observation 1 but not in Observation 2. When matching two sets of events, we need to consider all of the data recorded in potentially corresponding event records. In a team game, we typically have the video time of the event, the event type, the team performing the event, the particular player performing the event, the event location and the event outcome. These two sets of event records are usually set side by side in an Excel spreadsheet. The process involves identifying where an event has been recorded by one observer but not the other and then moving the other observer's data from this row onwards down one row to leave a gap for the missing event.

This matching process is typically manual and laborious, even if the data have been collected using a computerised system. We may have a

**Table 9.1** Sections of two Event Lists that have been matched revealing events identified by both observers as well as events identified by only a single observer

| Observation 1 | | | Observation 2 | | |
|---|---|---|---|---|---|
| Time (s) | Event | Player | Time (s) | Event | Player |
| 576.8 | Touch | BE | 576.8 | Touch | BE |
| 577.6 | Clearance | NB | 577.6 | Clearance | NB |
| 582.8 | Ball out of play | NULL | 582.1 | Ball out of play | NULL |
| | | | 591.2 | Throw in | WB |
| | | | 593.1 | Header | NS |
| | | | 593.8 | Ball out of play | NULL |
| 598.1 | Throw in | SK | 598.1 | Throw in | SK |
| 599.1 | Touch | JM | 599.1 | Touch | JM |
| 599.6 | Pass | JM | 599.6 | Pass | JM |
| 600.4 | Touch | WB | 600.4 | Touch | WB |
| 601.4 | Touch | WB | | | |
| 601.7 | Pass | WB | 601.7 | Pass | WB |
| 602.4 | Touch | JM | 602.4 | Touch | JM |

situation where an event record A in one observation could be matched with an event record B or an event record C in the other observation. The times at which the events are recorded might suggest event record A should be matched with event B while the other values in the event records might suggest event record A should be matches with event record C. There is no hard fast rule for prioritising time over other event data or vice versa. The analyst dealing with the reliability data needs to consider the extent to which the times disagree as well as any disagreements in the other values. Where the other values include event type, team, player 1, player 2, location and outcome, we could have situations where two event records agree for 0, 1, 2, 3, 4, 5 or all 6 of these variables. Consider a situation where an event record A in one observation is recorded at a time exactly halfway between the times at which event records B and C are recorded in the other observation. Now imagine that event records A and B also disagree on event type while event records A and C also disagree on outcome. We now need to consider the importance of the variables event type and outcome in deciding whether event record B or C could potentially correspond to event record A. Due to these philosophical considerations of the importance of event times and other event data, it is difficult to establish criteria for matching events that will be used within reliability studies of all systems where there are mismatching event lists.

If there are match periods (halves or quarters), a good first step is to identify corresponding blocks of records for each match period. The process of identifying event records recorded by a single observation, rather than both observations, can progress from beginning to end of the event lists or in the reverse order. The author has found a useful technique to help identify mismatching events in Excel which is to have an additional column showing the difference in event times. Where this jumps from being a fraction of a second to more than two seconds, we have a potential mismatch in the event records. These timing differences are inspected and if necessary, the rows of data for one observation are moved down to leave blank cells where no event record was recorded by one of the observations. This cutting and pasting of large numbers of rows can cause the additional time difference column to utilise times from outside the current row. Therefore, it is necessary to copy the time difference function from a row prior to the mismatch and paste into the remainder of the column to help identify the next mismatch that occurs.

There will be occasions where we see blank records for the first observation and occasions where we see blank records form the second observation. We may also have a situation where an event record that is only recorded by the first observation is immediately followed by one that is only recorded by the second observation (or vice versa). This might suggest that they could actually be matched. However, the disagreements in timings and/or the other variables recorded may be too great to justify matching them.

This all seems like a great deal of effort. It is! What readers need to remember is that this does not occur every time we use the system. This is only done within the reliability study of the system which is very important, especially if the system is to be used on many occasions in media, judging, coaching and or academic contexts.

## Exclusive events

Where we have a set of exclusively linked events, only one of these events can occur at a time. As one event is activated, it deactivates any other event in the set of events that may have been active up to that point in time. For example, in a racket sport we may have events representing states such as 'rally' and 'break' such that when we activate rally (or break) it deactivates the preceding break (or rally). Another example is

228

time motion analysis where we may have events representing seven different movement types: stationary, walking, backing, jogging, running shuffling and game-related activity. We will use this time-motion example to illustrate how to undertake a reliability assessment of a set of exclusively linked events in SportsCode.

This would typically work as an inter-operator reliability study where two independent operators tag the same video of a single player competing in a team game. Once this has been completed, we will have two timeline files to compare (t1 and t2). We have one problem to overcome, which is that both of the timelines have been created using the same Code Window and thus have the same row names. The way to overcome this is to make a copy of one of the timelines where we can use different row names. In this example we make a copy of the file t2 and call it t2copy. We select all seven rows in the file t2copy (stationary, walking, backing, jogging, running, shuffling and game-related) and duplicate them using **Rows → Duplicate selected rows**. This will create 7 new rows (stationary[1], walking[1], backing[1], jogging[1], running[1], shuffling[1] and game-related[1]) containing the same instances as the original rows. We can now delete the original 7 rows from t2copy.

Now we can merge the rows within t1 and t2copy into a merged timeline which we will call tmerged. This is done by opening the timeline files t1 and t2copy and selecting all seven rows in each file. We then use **File → Merge timeline windows** which creates a new timeline with all 14 rows copied into it which we save as tmerged.

We can use this reliability data to produce a value for O'Donoghue's (2005b) timed version of the kappa statistic. This determines the proportion of observation time where the observers agree on the activity being performed and adjusts this for the proportion of observation time where the observers would be expected to agree by guessing. The first thing we need to do with the newly created tmerged file is produce some new rows showing where the observers agree on the activity being performed. This is done for each of the seven movement types. Consider the rows representing where the two observers have recorded stationary activity (stationary and stationary[1]). We create a new row containing instances where the two observers agree that the player was stationary using **Row → Create new row** which causes a popup window to appear. In this popup window we advise that the new row will be called stationary_agreed, selecting the rows stationary and stationary[1] and applying the AND operator. This new row (stationary_agreed) only contains instances of stationary activity where there is some overlap between the instances recorded by the two observers.

Once we have done this for all seven movements we will have 21 rows of data as shown in Figure 9.2: seven for the movements recorded by observer 1, seven for the movements recorded by observer 2 and seven showing where the observers agree for each movement. We now use **File → Export → Instance Frequency** to save the timing data that we need to determine the kappa statistic. A popup window appears where we ensure that all rows are used and the output is sent to an Excel file which we can call timings.

The Excel file contains 21 rows of data; one for each row in the tmerged timeline. The Excel spreadsheet shows the number of instances (Count), the total of the times of instances (total time), the percentage of video time accounted for by these instances (%) and the mean time of an instance in the given row (Mean time). The total times can be transformed into the total number of seconds as described in Chapter 3. The 21 total times in seconds can now be used to calculate the kappa statistic.

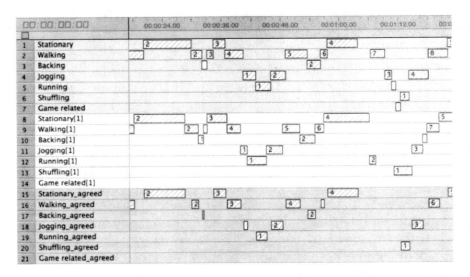

Figure 9.2 Timeline used for in assessing the reliability of exclusively linked events

In theory, the two observers should have started and ended their observations at exactly the same time within the video. However, this is not practical and so we use the longest of the two observation times. For each of the observers, we add the total time of the seven movements they have recorded. The longest of the two totals is noted, Total_Time. Remember that the whole video will contain some frames before the observation starts and after the observation finishes and so we need to determine Total_Time for the competitive performance observed.

We now add the totals for the seven agreed rows (stationary_agreed through to game related_agreed) giving Total_Agreed. We can now compute, $P_0$, which is needed for kappa as shown in Equation 9.1.

$$P_0 = \text{Total\_Agreed} / \text{Total\_Time} \tag{9.1}$$

To determine the proportion of time where the observers would be expected to agree by chance, $P_C$, we need to determine the expected amount of time the two observers would be expected to agree by chance for each movement type. Consider stationary movement where we will refer to the total time recorded by the two observers as Total_stationary and Total_stationary[1]. The expected time the two observers would be expected to agree by chance for this movement is given Equation 9.2.

$$\text{PC\_Stationary} = (\text{Total\_stationary} * \text{Total\_stationary[1]}) / \text{Total\_Time} \tag{9.2}$$

Once this is determined for each movement, the seven PC_movement totals are added to give PC_Total for the total amount of time the two observers would be expected to agree for any movement by guessing. We can now determine $P_C$ and kappa using Equations 9.3 and 9.4 respectively.

$$P_C = \text{PC\_Total} / \text{Total\_Time} \tag{9.3}$$

$$\text{Kappa} = (P_0 - P_C) / (1 - P_C) \tag{9.4}$$

## Timings

There are two types of timing data that can be derived from general purpose video analysis packages. These are the times at which events occur (or commence) and the duration of events. The accuracy that is necessary for any timings depends on how they are to be used. In many coaching situations, timing errors of up to three seconds can be tolerated where videos are tagged live during a match and video sequences are used in interactive debriefings. If the video sequences include a sufficient pre-roll (or lead time), then any time delay in recording events will not cause problems when viewing relevant video sequences later. This is a trade-off between the need for live data entry and accuracy of timing information. In the situation described, the priority is to have the video tagged live so that debriefing sessions can be prepared.

There are other situations where timing data are much more important and are not merely used to replay video sequences. For example, Greene *et al.* (2008) analysed touchdown times in international championship 400m hurdles races for scientific purposes. In this situation, the main priority was to have accurate timing information and the time taken to produce this was justified. Greene *et al.* used the Focus X2 system with publically available broadcast video of races recorded at 25 frames per second. This limited the precision of timings to the nearest 0.04s. Table 9.2 shows the timing errors made during the inter-observer reliability study of the method. There should be 88 values: eight athletes' touch-down times after ten hurdles as well as their finishing times. However, the video recording did not clearly show the athlete in lane 6 taking hurdles 2 and 3 meaning that there were only 86 timings recorded by each of the observers.

It is mathematically possible to determine mean absolute error (0.037s), 95 per cent limits of agreement (−0.007±0.111s), change in the mean (−0.007s) and standard error of measurement (0.040s). However, this is tenuous as the error values are multiples of 0.04s. Therefore, the reliability data shown in Table 9.2 should not be concealed from readers. In considering timing errors, we need to consider the use of the data. Are we interested in the specific touch down times or are we interested in times between different touch downs? If we are interested in the timings

Table 9.2 Inter-operator timing errors during the analysis of a 400m hurdles race

| Error | −0.20s | −0.16s | −0.12s | −0.08s | −0.04s | 0.00s | 0.04s | 0.08s | 0.12s | 0.16s | 0.20s |
|---|---|---|---|---|---|---|---|---|---|---|---|
| Frequency | 0 | 1 | 3 | 7 | 20 | 38 | 9 | 3 | 4 | 0 | 1 |

# 232

between touch downs at successive hurdles then the errors in these timings should be analysed as they come from two timing errors: one error at the first hurdle of the pair and one error at the second hurdle.

The main performance indicator used in Greene *et al.*'s research was the percentage increase in the time taken to do the second half of the race compared to the first half of the race. The time at halfway was taken as being 3/7 of the time between the touch down times at hurdles 5 and 6 because the 200m point is 15m after hurdle 5 and the hurdles are 35m apart. The values for this performance indicator during the reliability study are shown in Table 9.3. There are only eight pairs of values, which rules out the use of 95 per cent limits of agreement. Therefore, the reliability of this performance indicator can be described using the change in the mean (−0.04s) and the standard error of measurement (0.19s) which is sometimes also referred to as typical error.

## SPECIAL PURPOSE SYSTEMS

### Prozone MatchViewer

This section of the chapter describes reliability studies that have been done for special purpose systems used to analyse soccer. Prozone's MatchViewer system (Prozone, Leeds, UK) is an example of where mismatching events occur. The inter-operator reliability study involved

Table 9.3 Reliability of percentage increase in time taken to do second 200m of 400m hurdles race compared to the first 200m (%)

| Athlete (Lane) | Observer 1 | Observer 2 | Difference |
|---|---|---|---|
| 2 | 14.91 | 14.89 | 0.02 |
| 3 | 11.48 | 11.64 | −0.16 |
| 4 | 10.57 | 10.89 | −0.31 |
| 5 | 11.75 | 11.73 | 0.02 |
| 6 | 11.19 | 10.84 | 0.35 |
| 7 | 7.17 | 7.64 | −0.47 |
| 8 | 11.23 | 11.21 | 0.02 |
| 9 | 16.37 | 16.17 | 0.20 |
| Mean | 11.84 | 11.88 | −0.04 |
| SD | 2.79 | 2.62 | 0.27 |

determining which event records in one observation of a match corresponded to records in the other observation of the match (Bradley *et al.*, 2007). Each independent observation was carried out by an operator team rather than a single member of staff. Once the 2,552 events that had been recognised by both observers had been determined, the reliability study concentrated on disagreements for individual variables within event records. There were three types of data which were evaluated using different reliability statistics. First, there were nominal data such as event type, player and second player. The variable 'second player' was used for those event types involving two players such as passing. The reliability of these nominal variables was evaluated using the kappa statistic. The cross-tabulation of the frequencies of event types recorded by the two observations revealed occasions where the following values were confused:

- pass and cross;
- pass and touch;
- pass and offside;
- pass and clearance;
- tackle and touch.

There were 11 of the 2,552 occasions where the operator teams agreed that some event occurred where the operator teams disagreed over player performing the event. There were five further occasions where there was confusion between the two operator teams over who was the second player involved in an event. Some of these occasions were understandable perceptual errors. However, there was one occasion where the operator teams were confused between two players with very differing appearances. This was actually an example of a data entry error rather than a perceptual error because the buttons representing the two players were next to each other on the system interface set up for the match. These different types of error need to be explained in papers evaluating the reliability of systems.

The kappa value alone does not fully describe the level of inter-operator agreement and the types of error that can be made. Therefore, cross-tabulation of event type frequencies allows readers to make a more informed judgement of the level of reliability of the system. Where a paper is written specifically about the reliability of a system, this should appear in the results. Where the reliability study is not the main purpose of the

# 234

study but it is necessary to report the reliability of the data used, the cross-tabulated frequencies should be reported in an appendix while the kappa values are shown in the methods. A limitation of Bradley et al.'s study was that it only included the matching event records and, therefore, may have over-estimated system reliability.

The second type of data was event timings. The reliability of these was evaluated using mean absolute error of the timings of the 2,552 agreed events. The mean absolute error was 0.007s, but with this value being heavily influenced by the majority of occasions where the operator teams agreed exactly on the time of an event, it was also necessary to report that the agreement was within 0.1s for 95 per cent of the events.

The third type of data evaluated in the reliability study was event location, which was recorded as X and Y coordinates. Pythagoras' Theory was used to determine the distance between event locations entered by the two operator teams. Mean absolute error was used to summarise the location differences. The authors should have referred to this as mean error rather than mean absolute error because the equation from Pythagoras' Theory only produces positive values. The mean location error was 3.6m with 95 per cent of events being recorded within 8.5m by the two operator teams. The largest error of 70m was reported and explained by one occasion where the operator teams misjudging the orientation of the pitch diagram on which they were entering event locations. One operator team basically recorded the event as being in a diagonally opposite quadrant of the pitch to the one in which it actually occurred.

## Opta Sportsdata

The statistical techniques used by Bradley et al. (2007) to evaluate the reliability of Prozone's MatchViewer system are not the only ways in which the reliability of such data can be evaluated. One criticism of the approach is that it concentrated exclusively on the reliability of the raw data that were entered during the analysis of a soccer match rather than the reliability of output variables produced by the system. Liu et al. (2013) conducted an inter-operator agreement study for OPTA Sportsdata that combined analysis of reliability of input data as well as output information produced by the system. The kappa statistic was used to evaluate the reliability of event types. There were mismatching events and Liu et al. (2013) included all event records during their calculation of kappa, not just the agreed records. This study was more imaginative than Bradley *et al.*'s (2007) approach because separate kappa statistics were determined for the events performed by two teams in the match and separate kappa statistics were determined for the actions performed by goalkeepers and outfield players of each team. While event performed is a nominal variable at the data input stage, the frequency with which an event is performed by a player during the match is a ratio scale whole number. The frequencies of different events performed by individual players are of interest to coaches and analysts. Therefore, Liu *et al.* evaluated the reliability of these variables. This was done by determining the frequency for each event performed by each individual player according to the two independent observations. The mean, change in the mean and confidence limits for the change in the mean for the average player were then determined. Intra-class correlation coefficients and standardised typical errors were also determined for individual player event frequencies.

The change in the mean is simply the difference between the mean value of a numerical variable in the data recorded by two independent observations (Hopkins, 2000a). This is mathematically the same as the systematic bias used in 95 per cent limits of agreement (Bland and Altman, 1986). Typical error describes the error that is additional to the change in the mean in the same way that the random error component of 95 per cent limits of agreement is additional error to the systematic bias. In fact, typical error is directly proportional to random error. Random error is the standard deviation of the errors between two observations multiplied by 1.96. The multiplication by 1.96 is necessary because 68 per cent of normally distributed data are within one standard deviation of the mean for normally distributed data. Assuming the errors are normally distributed, 95 per cent of errors are within 1.96 standard deviations of the mean error. Thus 95 per cent limits of agreement are mean error ± 1.96 standard deviation of error. Hopkins (2000a) described 95 per cent limits of agreement as too stringent. The author of the current chapter has certainly experienced situations where the random error component of 95 per cent limits of agreement has been dismissed by reviewers as too large because they thought it was an average error. The 95 per cent limits of agreement represent a range of errors that only 5 per cent of errors are outside. Thus random error does not represent an average error. Hopkins (2000a) described typical error, s, as being the standard deviation of errors, $s_{diff}$, divided by $\sqrt{2}$. This was derived from the total variance of the differences in corresponding values between trials being the sum of variances representing the typical error in each trial, $s_{diff}^2 = s^2 + s^2$; hence, $s = s_{diff} / \sqrt{2}$. This represents 52 per cent of the spread of error values if the errors are normally distributed.

Standardised typical error is calculated using Equation 9.5 where TE is typical error, n1 and n2 are the number of values measured in each observation (usually n1 = n2) and s1 and s2 are the standard deviations of values measured in observations 1 and 2. Standardised typical error expresses typical error as a ratio of the variance within the data that is not down to typical error.

$$\text{Standardised TE} = \frac{TE}{\sqrt{\dfrac{((n1-1)s1^2+(n2-1)s2^2)}{(n1+n2-2)} - TE^2}} \tag{9.5}$$

Liu *et al.* (2013) found trivial disagreements for attack-related actions and total actions (standardised typical error < 0.2), small disagreements for defensive actions (standardised typical error = 0.21) and trivial to small typical errors for the frequencies of individual event types (standardised typical error < 0.6). Liu *et al.* (2013) used the criteria of Hopkins (2000b) to interpret the standardised typical error: less than 0.20 represents a trivial disagreement, 0.21–0.60 represents a small disagreement, 0.61–1.20 represents a moderate disagreement, 1.21–2.00 represents a large disagreement, 2.01–4.00 represents a very large disagreement and greater than 4.00 represents an extremely large disagreement.

Liu *et al.* (2013) also described the reliability of event timings between the independent teams that analysed the match used in their reliability study. They reported the mean ± standard deviation for event time. This could be done using absolute timing errors or signed timing errors. The advantage of the latter approach is that it gives an indication of systematic bias and random error components in the timings and is consistent with the change of the mean statistic used to assess reliability of event frequencies.

## Revisiting the data from Bradley *et al.* 2007

The reliability data for Prozone's MatchViewer system (Bradley *et al.*, 2007) is revisited here using the approach of Liu *et al.* (2013). There were 27 players in the match allowing means and standard deviations for individual player frequencies to be determined for different event types. Table 9.4 summarises the reliability data at individual player level for the seven most frequent events performed in the match and for the total number of events performed by individual players. All of the standardised typical errors are less than 0.2 which is interpreted as trivial disagreement between the two analysis teams. The Intra-class correlation coefficient can be determined using the reliability analysis facility of SPSS. This is accessed using **Analyse** → **Scale** → **Reliability**, clicking on the **Statistics** button and selecting Intraclass correlation coefficient.

**Prozone3**

The Prozone3 player tracking system (Prozone, Leeds, UK) uses image processing algorithms to track players during soccer matches. The process involves quality control personnel to verify players being followed where players may have been confused by the algorithms where the players have moved within close proximity of each other (Di Salvo *et al.*, 2009). A Prozone3 reliability study would require two independent copies of the system (software, hardware and human operators) to cover the same match. The costs and practical problems of implementing two copies of the system at a stadium for the purpose of a reliability study cannot be justified. Therefore, Prozone3 has been evaluated using validation studies rather than a reliability study. The thinking behind using a validation study is that if Prozone3 is consistent with some other

Table 9.4 Reliability of individual player event frequencies produced by Prozone's MatchViewer system

| Event | Obs Team 1 (mean±SD) | Obs Team 2 (mean±SD) | Change in the mean ± TE | Standardised TE | ICC |
|---|---|---|---|---|---|
| All events | 94.9±44.6 | 95.8±45.1 | 0.9±1.1 | 0.024 | 0.999 |
| Touch | 47.0±30.4 | 48.0±31.1 | 1.0±1.2 | 0.042 | 0.998 |
| Pass | 23.7±14.2 | 23.5±14.2 | −0.2±0.4 | 0.032 | 0.999 |
| Header | 5.7±5.2 | 5.7±5.4 | 0.0±0.2 | 0.051 | 0.997 |
| Tackle | 3.2±3.9 | 3.3±3.9 | 0.1±0.4 | 0.106 | 0.989 |
| Ball out of play | 2.8±14.6 | 2.8±14.8 | 0.0±0.1 | 0.009 | 1.000 |
| Clearance | 1.8±2.1 | 1.9±2.2 | 0.1±0.2 | 0.109 | 0.988 |
| Throw in | 1.8±4.0 | 1.8±4.1 | 0.0±0.1 | 0.033 | 0.999 |

acceptable measure of player movement then both methods may be reliable. If a method were unreliable, it would be applied inconsistently within an inter-operator reliability study and would, therefore, not be expected to be consistent with completely different methods producing the same variables. Two different validations studies have been conducted: an experimental validation against accurate electronic timing gates (Di Salvo et al., 2006) and a validation against a reliable human observational method (O'Donoghue and Robinson, 2009).

Di Salvo et al. (2006) validated Prozone3 against data recorded by electronic timing gates during a stadium test where six players performed a series of planned runs of known routes and distances. The planned runs were 15m sprints, 20m runs with a 90° turn in the middle, a 50m run with the first 30m being in a straight line and the last 20m following a curved path, and a 60m straight line run controlled by audio pacing signals. Correlations were used to show relative reliability while typical error and coefficient of variation were used to describe absolute reliability. There was a good strength of absolute and relative agreement between the speeds determined from the electronic timings and the speeds determined from player locations recorded by Prozone3. Di Salvo et al. (2009) reanalysed the data from Di Salvo et al.'s (2006) stadium study using mixed model repeated measures ANOVA tests and percentage coefficient of variation. The coefficient of variation for the pooled data was 0.4 per cent which is further evidence that the velocities derived from the timed player locations recorded by Prozone3 are highly accurate.

The controlled experiment conducted by Di Salvo et al. (2006) had many advantages over validating Prozone against an approach using human observers with real match data. In particular, the electronic timing gates are more accurate and reliable than human observation. However, approaches using real match data also have advantages over controlled experiments (Carling et al., 2008). Movements performed during matches are logically more representative of the game and are performed in an environment where other players are competing rather than being performed in isolation. Therefore, O'Donoghue and Robinson (2009) undertook a case study to validate a single player's movement data recorded by Prozone3 against a human observation approach that recorded path changes as well as where the player made transitions between different areas of the pitch. This required the player to be filmed for the full duration of the match.

Path changes were recorded when movement during the 1s before and/or 1s after the point of path change was performed at 2 m.s⁻¹ or faster. There were three types of path change of interest: sharp path changes to the left, sharp path changes to the right and V-cuts. The sharp path changes to the left (or right) were defined as any movement where the direction changed by between 45° and 135° to the left (or right). A V-cut was where the player changed direction between 135° to the left and 135° to the right going in the opposite direction to the direction travelled before the path change. An inter-operator agreement study revealed the human observation of these path changes had a good strength of agreement (κ = 0.71). There were expected errors due to the difficulty for human operators recognising movement speeds close to 2 m.s⁻¹, path changes of about 135° being on the border of a sharp path change and a V-cut, path changes of about 45° being on the border of a sharp path change no path change being made and some path changes being confused with movements in arced directions. Having established the level of agreement between the two human observers, the path changes they located were compared with those recognised by an algorithm applied to Prozone3 data. This revealed a moderate strength of agreement between the data derived from the human observers and the data derived from Prozone3 (the κ value was 0.41 between Prozone and each of the two human observers).

The areas of the pitch were analysed using the 17 areas shown in Figure 9.3 because line markings were visible and the grass had been cut in a manner that assisted the identification of pitch areas. The dimensions of the pitch were known to be 105m long and 66m wide. The Prozone data were processed in Microsoft Excel to determine the times at which the player moved from one area to another. Two independent observers watched the video recording of the player's performance recording the times at which the player moved from one pitch area to another. The two observers agreed on the times at which areas were entered within 1s for 99.0 per cent of area entries recorded. The times of area entries derived from Prozone3 data were within 1s of those recorded by the two human observers for 95.7 per cent and 96.7 per cent of area entries. There were three sources of disagreement between Prozone3 and the human observers. First, there were occasions where the player briefly moved through the corner of an area. Second, there were occasions when the player moved into the area momentarily. Third, there were occasions where the player moved less than 1m into the area.

240

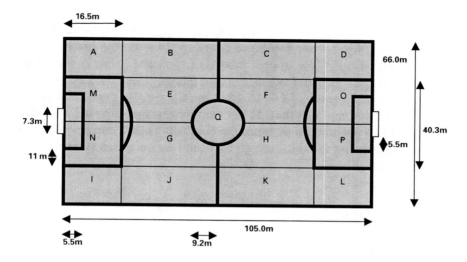

Figure 9.3 Areas of the pitch used in O'Donoghue and Robinson's validation of Prozone3 against human observation

The two types of data (path changes and entries into different areas of the pitch) do not cover all movements made by the players. However, a process of inductive reasoning can be used to argue the validity of the system. If the times at which path changes are made can be identified, then this provides evidence that relative changes in player location can be recognised by Prozone3. Similarly, if the times at which players enter different areas can be recognised by Prozone3 then there is evidence that player location can be recognised. Given that locations are timed correctly over the course of the match, we can argue that distances covered and movement speeds can also be determined from this data.

Although a reliability study involving two installations of the Prozone3 system at a stadium has been ruled out as impractical, intra- and inter-operator agreement studies have been carried out on the manual verification process applied by quality control personnel involved in the system (Di Salvo et al., 2009). The movement of two players that had been recorded by the automated element of the system was verified by two independent quality control staff on two occasions each giving four sets of data for the purpose of reliability assessment. The data were organised into 5 minute 'data bins' to allow the coefficient of variation to be determined for distance covered at different speed ranges. The coefficients of variation between observers were largest for distances when sprinting (faster than 25.2 km.h⁻¹, CV = 6.5 per cent), high speed running (19.8 to 25.2 km.h⁻¹, CV = 4.8 per cent) and running (14.4 to 19.8 km.h⁻¹, CV = 3.7 per cent) with the lowest coefficients of variation between observers being for distance covered when walking (slower than 7.2 km.h⁻¹, CV = 1.5 per cent) and jogging (7.2 to 14.4 km.h⁻¹, CV = 2.0 per cent). The coefficients of variation of less than 10 per cent for distance covered sprinting and less than 5 per cent for distance covered using other movements were interpreted as being reliable enough for coaching purposes and scientific applications.

## WEB-BASED DATA

### Match statistics

Match statistics are provided on official tournament websites. For example, the official sites of the four Grand Slam tennis tournaments contain various match statistics that are used for media, coaching and scientific purposes. When using the data for any serious purpose, it is essential to demonstrate the validity and reliability of the data. Validity can be argued from the importance and relevance of the particular match statistics provided on the internet. Validity can be compromised if the variables used have vague or non-existent definitions. For example, what counts as an unforced error in tennis? If this is left undefined, then it may be have been judged subjectively by those gathering the data for the official tournament internet sites. This lack of objectivity can lessen the reliability of a performance indicator such as the percentage of points where a player makes an unforced error. A variable has to be reliable in order to be valid. There may also be situations where there are detailed definitions of the events recorded during matches but these are not made available to the users of the official tournament internet sites.

There are some variables that should be commonly understood. For example, the number of points where the first serve was in, the number of points won when the first serve was in, the number of second serve points, the number of second serve points that were won, the number of break points played and the number of break points won. These variables were used in a study of break point performance compared to non-break point performance when receiving serve (Knight and O'Donoghue, 2012).

Despite the apparent obvious classification of service, score-line state and whether a point was won or not, Knight and O'Donoghue (2012) still validated these variables against values recorded from video observation of a sample of four matches; one from each Grand Slam tournament. They described this as a quasi-estimation of the reliability of the data provided on the internet. There was complete agreement between the values provided on the internet and those derived from video observation for all of the variables used in all 4 matches.

Two more problematic variables are the percentage of points where a player goes to the net and the percentage of points won when a player goes to the net. These both rely on identifying individual net points correctly. The official internet sites of the Grand Slam tennis tournaments provide data for the number of net points played and won by each player. However, there is no definition of what counts as a net point on any of these internet sites. The author of the current chapter has had private communication with individuals who have gathered data for these websites about the training they received and the guidance they were given about identifying net points. There does appear to be an element of subjectivity in deciding how far forward from the baseline counts as being at the net. For the purpose of this chapter, we will use this as an example of quasi-estimation of reliability. The author watched 20 sets from nine women's singles tennis matches played at the Australian and US Open tennis tournaments. Therefore, there were 40 different player performances at individual set level. The author applied two definitions of net points during the video observation.

Definition 1: A player plays a net point when they cross into either service box when either player still has to play at least one more shot in the point.

Definition 2: A player plays a net point when they cross into either service box before the point has ended according to the rules of tennis. The point ends when a ball strikes the net, lands out or bounces twice without being retrieved by a player.

The first definition is close to how O'Donoghue and Ingram (2001) classified net points, except in this example, the point can be classified as a net point for one or both of the players. The second definition is close to the guidance given to analysts working at the Grand Slam tournaments. Table 9.5 shows the data recorded using these two definitions as well as the corresponding values provided on the official tournament websites.

Table 9.5 Net points played and won according to two video observation methods and the official tournament websites

| Player site | Video Observation Definition 1 | | | Video Observation Definition 2 | | | Official Tournament Internet | | |
|---|---|---|---|---|---|---|---|---|---|
| | Net Pts Won | Net Pts | Total Pts | Net Pts Won | Net Pts | Total Pts | Net Pts Won | Net Pts | Total Pts |
| Radwanska A | 6 | 8 | 85 | 7 | 9 | 85 | 6 | 7 | 85 |
| Torro-Flor | 7 | 10 | 85 | 11 | 14 | 85 | 11 | 14 | 85 |
| Robson | 1 | 1 | 50 | 2 | 3 | 50 | 2 | 3 | 50 |
| Garcia | 0 | 1 | 50 | 3 | 4 | 50 | 3 | 4 | 50 |
| Robson | 1 | 1 | 84 | 2 | 3 | 84 | 2 | 2 | 84 |
| Garcia | 3 | 3 | 84 | 5 | 7 | 84 | 4 | 6 | 84 |
| Robson | 0 | 1 | 46 | 0 | 1 | 46 | 0 | 1 | 46 |
| Li | 1 | 1 | 46 | 5 | 6 | 46 | 5 | 5 | 46 |
| Robson | 2 | 3 | 73 | 3 | 4 | 73 | 3 | 4 | 73 |
| Li | 2 | 2 | 73 | 4 | 4 | 73 | 4 | 4 | 73 |
| Cornet | 1 | 2 | 50 | 3 | 4 | 50 | 2 | 3 | 50 |
| Kohler | 0 | 0 | 50 | 1 | 2 | 50 | 3 | 4 | 4 |
| Cornet | 1 | 2 | 84 | 1 | 2 | 63 | 2 | 2 | 63 |
| Kohler | 3 | 4 | 84 | 3 | 5 | 63 | 4 | 6 | 63 |
| Petrova | 3 | 3 | 52 | 3 | 4 | 52 | 3 | 3 | 52 |
| Szavay | 2 | 2 | 52 | 2 | 3 | 52 | 2 | 3 | 52 |
| Petrova | 3 | 4 | 69 | 3 | 8 | 69 | 5 | 8 | 69 |
| Szavay | 2 | 3 | 69 | 2 | 4 | 69 | 2 | 4 | 69 |
| Szavay | 3 | 6 | 42 | 3 | 7 | 42 | 3 | 7 | 42 |
| Kuznetzova | 1 | 1 | 42 | 3 | 4 | 42 | 2 | 3 | 42 |
| Szavay | 3 | 7 | 62 | 3 | 8 | 62 | 3 | 7 | 62 |
| Kuznetzova | 2 | 3 | 62 | 4 | 6 | 62 | 5 | 6 | 62 |
| Halep | 4 | 4 | 60 | 4 | 5 | 60 | 3 | 4 | 60 |
| Watson | 2 | 2 | 60 | 2 | 3 | 60 | 2 | 4 | 60 |
| Halep | 4 | 5 | 67 | 4 | 6 | 67 | 4 | 5 | 67 |
| Watson | 1 | 2 | 67 | 1 | 2 | 67 | 1 | 1 | 67 |
| Halep | 5 | 6 | 47 | 5 | 6 | 47 | 5 | 6 | 47 |
| Watson | 0 | 0 | 47 | 0 | 0 | 47 | 0 | 0 | 47 |
| Williams S | 2 | 7 | 71 | 2 | 7 | 71 | 2 | 5 | 71 |
| Azarenka | 1 | 1 | 71 | 3 | 3 | 71 | 2 | 2 | 71 |
| Williams S | 1 | 3 | 83 | 3 | 6 | 83 | 1 | 5 | 83 |
| Azarenka | 5 | 6 | 83 | 6 | 7 | 83 | 7 | 8 | 83 |
| Williams S | 0 | 2 | 46 | 1 | 3 | 46 | 1 | 3 | 46 |
| Azarenka | 1 | 4 | 46 | 1 | 4 | 46 | 1 | 5 | 46 |
| Azarenka | 1 | 2 | 69 | 3 | 4 | 69 | 3 | 4 | 69 |
| Li | 1 | 2 | 69 | 3 | 5 | 69 | 2 | 5 | 69 |
| Azarenka | 3 | 5 | 66 | 5 | 7 | 66 | 5 | 8 | 66 |
| Li | 2 | 4 | 66 | 3 | 5 | 66 | 3 | 5 | 66 |
| Azarenka | 0 | 2 | 57 | 1 | 3 | 57 | 0 | 2 | 57 |
| Li | 1 | 1 | 57 | 2 | 2 | 57 | 1 | 1 | 57 |

One thing that should be immediately apparent to readers is that we are dealing with fractions, especially when considering the percentage of net points that are won. Consider Laura Robson's second set against Li Na where she won 2/3 (66.7 per cent) net points according to one method and 3/4 (75.0 per cent) according to the other two methods. This has probably resulted from one error where a won point was considered to be a net point by two of the methods but not the other. Table 9.5 also shows that the frequencies recorded according to Definition 2 are closer to those provided on the official tournament internet sites. Therefore, the quasi-estimation of reliability only compares Definition 2 with the internet data. The raw frequencies in Table 9.5 are used to determine the percentage of net points won and the percentage of points that are net points. These values are shown in Table 9.6. There was one set performance where the player (Heather Watson) did not play any net points according to Definition 2 or the internet data. This means that the percentage of net points that were won is undefined for this case.

The standard deviations of the differences in values between two methods are divided by $\sqrt{2}$ to give the typical error for the given variable. The percentage of points that are net points has a typical error of 0.97 per cent and a standardised typical error of 0.19, which represents a trivial disagreement between video observation and the internet data. The percentage of net points that are won has a typical error of 12.25 per cent and a standardised typical error of 0.57, which represents a small disagreement between video observation and the internet data. There is an intra-class correlation coefficient of 0.931 for the percentage of points that are net points and 0.756 for the percentage of net points that are won. Whether users can accept the interpretation of standardised typical error proposed by Hopkins (2000b) depends on the analytical goals of the study being done. The standard deviation of differences between the two methods for the percentage of net points that are won is 17.3 per cent which equates to a random error of 33.96 per cent. This does seem very high in relation to the means of 62.8 per cent from video observation and 66.6 per cent from the internet data. However, when one considers the possibility of one method recording 0/1 = 0 per cent of net points won and an alternative method recording 1/2 = 50 per cent of net points won, it is actually surprising the random error figure is not higher. Random error represents the spread of errors about the systematic bias of −3.8 per cent that only 5 per cent of errors would be outside (Atkinson and Nevill, 1998).

Table 9.6 Reliability of percentage versions of net point variables

| Player | Percentage of points that were net points | | | Percentage of net points that were won | | |
| | Definition 2 | Internet | Difference | Definition 2 | Internet | Difference |
| --- | --- | --- | --- | --- | --- | --- |
| Radwanska A | 10.6 | 8.2 | 2.4 | 77.8 | 85.7 | −7.9 |
| Torro-Flor | 16.5 | 16.5 | 0.0 | 78.6 | 78.6 | 0.0 |
| Robson | 6.0 | 6.0 | 0.0 | 66.7 | 66.7 | 0.0 |
| Garcia | 8.0 | 8.0 | 0.0 | 75.0 | 75.0 | 0.0 |
| Robson | 3.6 | 2.4 | 1.2 | 66.7 | 100.0 | −33.3 |
| Garcia | 8.3 | 7.1 | 1.2 | 71.4 | 66.7 | 4.8 |
| Robson | 2.2 | 2.2 | 0.0 | 0.0 | 0.0 | 0.0 |
| Li | 13.0 | 10.9 | 2.2 | 83.3 | 100.0 | −16.7 |
| Robson | 5.5 | 5.5 | 0.0 | 75.0 | 75.0 | 0.0 |
| Li | 5.5 | 5.5 | 0.0 | 100.0 | 100.0 | 0.0 |
| Cornet | 8.0 | 6.0 | 2.0 | 75.0 | 66.7 | 8.3 |
| Kohler | 4.0 | 8.0 | −4.0 | 50.0 | 75.0 | −25.0 |
| Cornet | 3.2 | 2.4 | 0.8 | 50.0 | 100.0 | −50.0 |
| Kohler | 7.9 | 7.1 | 0.8 | 60.0 | 66.7 | −6.7 |
| Petrova | 7.7 | 5.8 | 1.9 | 75.0 | 100.0 | −25.0 |
| Szavay | 5.8 | 5.8 | 0.0 | 66.7 | 66.7 | 0.0 |
| Petrova | 11.6 | 11.6 | 0.0 | 37.5 | 62.5 | −25.0 |
| Szavay | 5.8 | 5.8 | 0.0 | 50.0 | 50.0 | 0.0 |
| Szavay | 16.7 | 16.7 | 0.0 | 42.9 | 42.9 | 0.0 |
| Kuznetzova | 9.5 | 7.1 | 2.4 | 75.0 | 66.7 | 8.3 |
| Szavay | 12.9 | 11.3 | 1.6 | 37.5 | 42.9 | −5.4 |
| Kuznetzova | 9.7 | 9.7 | 0.0 | 66.7 | 83.3 | −16.7 |
| Halep | 8.3 | 6.7 | 1.7 | 80.0 | 75.0 | 5.0 |
| Watson | 5.0 | 6.7 | −1.7 | 66.7 | 50.0 | 16.7 |
| Halep | 9.0 | 7.5 | 1.5 | 66.7 | 80.0 | −13.3 |
| Watson | 3.0 | 1.5 | 1.5 | 50.0 | 100.0 | −50.0 |
| Halep | 12.8 | 12.8 | 0.0 | 83.3 | 83.3 | 0.0 |
| Watson | 0.0 | 0.0 | 0.0 | | | |
| Williams S | 9.9 | 7.0 | 2.8 | 28.6 | 40.0 | −11.4 |
| Azarenka | 4.2 | 2.8 | 1.4 | 100.0 | 100.0 | 0.0 |
| Williams S | 7.2 | 6.0 | 1.2 | 50.0 | 20.0 | 30.0 |
| Azarenka | 8.4 | 9.6 | −1.2 | 85.7 | 87.5 | −1.8 |
| Williams S | 6.5 | 6.5 | 0.0 | 33.3 | 33.3 | 0.0 |
| Azarenka | 8.7 | 10.9 | −2.2 | 25.0 | 20.0 | 5.0 |
| Azarenka | 5.8 | 5.8 | 0.0 | 75.0 | 75.0 | 0.0 |
| Li | 7.2 | 7.2 | 0.0 | 60.0 | 40.0 | 20.0 |
| Azarenka | 10.6 | 12.1 | −1.5 | 71.4 | 62.5 | 8.9 |
| Li | 7.6 | 7.6 | 0.0 | 60.0 | 60.0 | 0.0 |
| Azarenka | 5.3 | 3.5 | 1.8 | 33.3 | 0.0 | 33.3 |
| Li | 3.5 | 1.8 | 1.8 | 100.0 | 100.0 | 0.0 |
| Mean | 8.4 | 7.1 | 0.5 | 62.8 | 66.6 | −3.8 |
| SD | 6.2 | 3.7 | 1.4 | 21.9 | 27.4 | 17.3 |

The reliability study has been conducted on set data, which is important if individual set data are to be used in the main scientific study. However, if full match data are to be used then we might expect smaller typical error values due to larger numbers of points avoiding large percentage disagreements between small fractions such as 0/1 and 1/2.

## SUMMARY

This chapter has illustrated some of the pre-processing tasks that need to be done during reliability studies, for examples converting times into decimal numbers (total seconds), exporting data from commercial packages and dealing with mismatching event lists. Both general purpose and special purpose systems have many different types of data that are evaluated using different reliability statistics. For example, the reliability of player location is evaluated using mean location difference. An issue in published reliability studies of special purpose systems, such as Opta Sportsdata and Prozone's MatchViewer, is whether to analyse the reliability of the raw data that have been gathered or the reliability of output information that is produced. The approach of Liu *et al.* (2013) is recommended as it analyses the reliability of raw input data as well as the frequencies that would be output for individual players. The standardised typical error relates typical error to the variability found in the given variables and has a means of determining the seriousness of any disagreements between observations. Some systems such as Prozone3 cannot be installed twice at the same stadium to allow a reliability study to compare two independent sets of data produced by the same type of system. There are also data provided on internet sites that cannot be evaluated for inter-operator agreement because internet users may not have access to the systems used to collect the data. In cases like these, quasi-estimation of reliability is done by validating system or internet data against some alternative method that can be applied by researchers.

# REFERENCES

Altman, D. G. (1991) *Practical Statistics for Medical Research*, London: Chapman & Hall.

Anderson, D. R., Sweeney, D. J. and Williams, T. A. (1994) *Introduction to Statistics: Concepts and Applications*, 3rd edn, Minneapolis/St Paul: West Publishing Company.

Atkinson, G. and Nevill, A. M. (1998) 'Statistical methods for addressing measurement error (reliability) in variables relevant to sports medicine', *Sports Medicine*, 26: 217–38.

Bangsbo, J. and Peitersen, B. (2002) *Defensive Soccer Tactics: How to Stop Players and Teams from Scoring*, Champaign, IL: Human Kinetics.

Bangsbo, J. and Peitersen, B. (2004) *Offensive Soccer Tactics: How to Control Possession and Score More Goals*, Champaign, IL: Human Kinetics.

Bartlett, R. M. (2004) 'Artificial intelligence in performance analysis', *International Journal of Performance Analysis in Sport*, 4(2): 4–19.

Bland, J. M. and Altman, D. G. (1986) 'Statistical methods for assessing the agreement between two methods of clinical measurement', *Lancet*, I: 307–10.

Bloomfield, J., Jonsson, G. K., Polman, R., Houlahan, K. and O'Donoghue, P. (2005) 'Temporal pattern analysis and its applicability in soccer', in L. Anolli, S. Duncan, M. Magnusson and G. Riva (eds), *The Hidden Structure of Social Interaction: From Genomics to Culture Patterns* (pp. 51–70), Amsterdam: IOS Press.

Borrie, A., Jonsson, G. K. and Magnusson, M. S. (2002) 'Temporal pattern analysis and its applicability in sport: An explanation and exemplar data', *Journal of Sports Sciences*, 20: 845–52.

Bradley, P., O'Donoghue, P. G., Wooster, B. and Tordoff, P. (2007) 'The reliability of ProZone MatchViewer: a video-based technical performance analysis system', *International Journal of Performance Analysis in Sport*, 7: 117–29.

Bugaets, A. N., Vostroknutov, E. P. and Vostroknutova, A. I. (1991) 'Artificial intelligence methods in geological forecasting', *Mathematical Geology*, 23: 9–13.

Carling, C. and Bloomfield, J. (2013) 'Time-motion analysis', in T. McGarry, P. G.

O'Donoghue and J. Sampaio (eds), *Routledge Handbook of Sports Performance Analysis* (pp. 283–96), London: Routledge.

Carling, C., Bloomfield, J., Nelson, L. and Reilly, T. (2008) 'The role of motion analysis in elite soccer: contemporary performance measurement techniques and work rate data', *Sports Medicine*, 38: 839–62.

Cohen, L., Manion, L. and Morrison, K. (2011) *Research Methods in Education*, 7th edn, London: Routledge.

Daniel, J. (2003) *The Complete Guide to Soccer Systems and Tactics*, Spring City, PA: Reedswain Publishing.

Davidson, F. (1996) *Principles of Statistical Data Handling*, Thousand Oaks, CA: Sage Publications.

Di Salvo, V., Collins, A., McNeill, B. and Cardinale, M. (2006) 'Validation of Prozone®: a new video-based performance analysis system', *International Journal of Performance Analysis of Sport*, 6(1): 108–19.

Di Salvo, V., Gregson, W., Atkinson, G., Tordoff, P. and Drust, B. (2009) 'Analysis of high intensity activity in Premier League soccer', *International Journal of Sports Medicine*, 30: 205–12.

Diamantopoulos, A. and Schlegelmilch, B. B. (1997) *Taking the Fear Out of Data Analysis*, London: The Dryden Press.

Dijk, J. (2011) 'Training and performance management in the top', World Congress of Science and Football 7, Book of Abstracts (p. 32), Nagoya, Japan, 26–30 May.

Duarte, R., Araújo, D., Davids, K., Folgado, H., Marques, P. and Ferreira, A. (2011) 'In search of dyanmic patterns of team tactical behaviours during competitive football performance', World Congress of Science and Football 7, Book of Abstracts (p. 114), Nagoya, Japan, 26–30 May.

Endsley, M. R. and Jones, D. G. (2004) *Designing for Situation Awareness: An Approach to User-Centred Design*, New York: Taylor & Francis Group.

Fallowfield, J. L., Hale, B. J. and Wilkinson, D. M. (2005) *Using Statistics in Sport and Exercise Science Research*, Chichester: Lotus Publishing.

Few, S. (2006) *Information Dashboard Design: The Effective Visual Communication of Data*, Sebastopol, CA: O'Reilly Media, Inc.

Few, S. (2013) *Information Dashboard Design: Displaying Data for At-a-glance Monitoring*, Burlingame, CA: Analytics Press.

Fonseca, S., Milho, J., Travassos, B., Araújo, D. and Lopes, A. (2013) 'Measuring spatial interaction behaviour in team sports using superimposed Voronoi diagrams', *International Journal of Performance Analysis in Sport*, 13: 179–89.

Franks, I. M. and Miller, G. (1991) 'Training coaches to observe and remember', *Journal of Sports Sciences*, 9: 285–97

Frawley, W. J., Piatetsky-Shapiro, G. W. J. and Matheus, C. J. (1991) 'Knowledge discovery in databases: an overview', in G. Piatetsky-Shapiro and W. Frawley (eds) *Knowledge Discovery in Databases* (pp. 1–27), Cambridge, MA: AAAI/MIT Press.

Frencken, W., Lemmink, K., Delleman, N. and Visscher, C. (2011) 'Oscillations of centroid position and surface area of soccer teams in small-sided games', *European Journal of Sport Science*, 11: 215–23.

Gomez, M. A., Lagos-Pe as, C. and Pollard, R. (2013) 'Situational variables', in T.

McGarry, P. G. O'Donoghue and J. Sampaio (eds), *Routledge Handbook of Sports Performance Analysis* (pp. 259–69), London: Routledge.

Graham, A. (1991) *Handling Data*, Milton Keynes: Open University Press.

Greene, D., Leyshon, W. and O'Donoghue, P. G. (2008) 'Elite male 400m hurdle tactics are influenced by race leader', World Congress of Performance Analysis of Sport 8, Magdeburg, 3–6 September.

Gréhaigne, J. F., Bouthier, D. and David, B. (1997) 'A method to analyse attacking moves in soccer', in T. Reilly, J. Bangsbo and M. Hughes (eds) *Sciences and Football III* (pp. 258–64) London: E. & F.N. Spon.

Hargreaves, A. and Bate, R. (2010) *Skills and Strategies for Soccer Coaching: The Complete Soccer Coaching Manual*, 2nd edn, Champaign, IL: Human Kinetics.

Healey, C. G., Booth, K. S. and Enns, J. T. (1996) 'High-speed visual estimation using preattentive processing', *ACM Transactions on Computer-Human Interaction*, 3(2): 107–35.

Hinton, P. R. (2004) *Statistics Explained*, 2nd edn, London: Routledge.

Hopkins, W. G. (2000a) 'Measurement of reliability in sports medicine and science', *Sports Medicine*, 30: 1–15.

Hopkins, W. G. (2000b) 'Reliability for consecutive pair of trials (Excel Spreadsheet)', in 'A new view of statistics', Sportsci.org: Internet Society for Sport Science. sportsci.org/resource/stats/xrely.xls

Hughes, C. (1994) *The Football Association Coaching Book of Soccer Tactics and Skills*, Harpenden: Queen Anne Press.

Hughes, M. and Franks, I. M. (eds) (2004a) *Notational Analysis of Sport: Systems for Better Coaching and Performance in Sport*, 2nd edn, London: Routledge.

Hughes, M. and Franks, I. M. (2004b) 'How to develop a notation system', In M. Hughes and I.M. Franks (eds), *Notational Analysis of Sport: Systems for Better Coaching and Performance in Sport*, 2nd edn (pp. 118–40), London: Routledge.

Hughes, M. and Franks, I. M. (2008) *The Essentials of Performance Analysis of Sport*, London: Routledge.

Hughes, M., Cooper, S. M. and Nevill, A. (2004) 'Analysis of notation data: reliability', in M. Hughes and I. M. Franks (eds), *Notational Analysis of Sport: Systems for Better Coaching and Performance in Sport*, 2nd edn (pp. 189–204). London: Routledge.

James, N., Jones, N. M. P. and Hollely, C. (2002) 'Reliability of selected performance analysis systems in football and rugby', Proceedings of the 4th International Conference on Methods and Techniques in Behavioural Research, Amsterdam, pp. 116–18.

Kirk-Smith, M. (1998) 'Psychological issues in questionnaire based research', *Journal of the Market Research Society*, 40: 223–6.

Knight, G. and O'Donoghue, P. G. (2012) 'The probability of winning break points in Grand Slam men's singles tennis', *European Journal of Sports Science*, 12(6): 462–8.

Laird, P. and Waters, L. (2008) 'Eye-witness recollection of sports coaches', *International Journal of Performance Analysis of Sport*, 8(1): 76–84.

Lamb, P. and Bartlett, R. (2013) 'Neural networks for analysing sports techniques', in T. McGarry, P. G. O'Donoghue and J. Sampaio (eds) *Routledge Handbook of Sports Performance Analysis* (pp. 225–36), London: Routledge.

250

Lames, M. and Siegle, M. (2011) 'Positional data in game sports – validation and practical impact', keynote address, 8th International Symposium of Computer Science in Sport, Shanghai, China. 21–24 September.

Lames, M., Siegle, M. and O'Donoghue, P. G. (2013) 'An exploratory evaluation of measures of space creation and restriction in soccer', in D. Peters and P. G. O'Donoghue (eds) *Performance Analysis of Sport IX* (pp. 275–81), London: Routledge.

Lames, M., Cordes, O. and Walter, F. (2009) 'Relative phase and oscillations in football', paper presented at the 3rd International Workshop of the International Society of Performance Analysis of Sport, Lincoln, 6–7 April.

Lapham, A. C. and Bartlett, R. (1995) 'The use of artificial intelligence in the analysis of sports performance: a review of applications in human gait analysis and future directions for sports biomechanics', *Journal of Sports Sciences*, 13: 229–37.

Lapresa, D., Anguera, M. T., Alsasua, R., Arana, J. and Garzón, B. (2013), 'Comparative analysis of T-patterns using real time data and simulated data by assignment of conventional durations: the construction of efficacy in children's basketball', *International Journal of Sports Performance Analysis*, 13: 321–39.

Lemminck, K. A. P. M. and Frencken, W. G. P. (2011), 'Tactical match analysis in soccer: new perspectives?', World Congress of Science and Football 7, Book of Abstracts (p. 22), Nagoya, Japan, 26–30 May.

Leser, R. and Roemer, K. (2014) 'Computer video systems', in A.Baca (ed.) *Sports Informatics*, London: Routledge.

Lewis, M. (2003). *Moneyball: The Art of Winning an Unfair Game*. New York: W.W. Norton & Company.

Liu, H., Hopkins, W., Gómez, M. A. and Molinuevo, J. S. (2013) 'Inter-operator reliability of live football match statistics from OPTA Sportsdata', *International Journal of Performance Analysis in Sport*, 13: 803–21.

McGarry, T., O'Donoghue, P. G. and Sampaio, J. (2013), *Routledge Handbook of Sports Performance Analysis*, London: Routledge.

Magnusson, M. S. (2000) 'Discovering hidden time patterns in behavior: T-patterns and their detection', *Behavior Research Methods, Instruments and Computers*, 32(1): 93–110.

Martin, S. (2011) 'Virtual world in educational research', in L. Cohen, L. Manion and K. Morrison (eds.) *Research Methods in Education*, 7th edn (pp. 362–74), London: Routledge.

O'Donoghue, P. G. (2003) 'The effect of scoreline on elite tennis strategy: a cluster analysis', *Journal of Sports Sciences*, 21: 284–5.

O'Donoghue, P. G. (2005a) 'The role of simulation in sports tournament design for game sport', *International Journal of Computer Science in Sport*, 4(2): 14–27.

O'Donoghue, P. G. (2005b) 'An algorithm to use the kappa statistic to establish reliability of computerised time-motion analysis systems', 5th International Symposium of Computer Science in Sport, Book of Abstracts (p. 49), Hvar, Croatia, 25–28 May.

O'Donoghue, P. G. (2006a) 'Elite tennis strategy during tie-breaks', in H. Dancs,

M. Hughes and P. G. O'Donoghue (eds) *Performance Analysis of Sport 7* (pp. 654–60), Cardiff: CPA Press, UWIC.

O'Donoghue, P. G. (2006b) 'The effectiveness of satisfying the assumptions of predictive modelling techniques: an exercise in predicting the FIFA World Cup 2006', *International Journal of Computing Science in Sport*, 5(2): 5–16.

O'Donoghue, P. G. (2010) *Research Methods for Sports Performance Analysis*, London: Routledge.

O'Donoghue, P. G. (2011) 'Automatic recognition of balance and in soccer defences using player displacement data', keynote address, 8th International Symposium of Computer Science in Sport, Shanghai, 21–24 September.

O'Donoghue, P. G. (2012) *Statistics for Sport and Exercise Studies: An Introduction*, London: Routledge.

O'Donoghue, P. G. (2015) *An Introduction to Performance Analysis of Sport*, London: Routledge.

O'Donoghue, P. G. and Brown, E. J. (2009) 'Sequences of service points and the misperception of momentum in elite tennis', *International Journal of Performance Analysis in Sport*, 9(1): 113–27.

O'Donoghue, P. G. and Ingram, B. (2001) 'A notational analysis of elite tennis strategy', *Journal of Sports Sciences*, 19: 107–15.

O'Donoghue, P. G. and Longville, J. (2004) 'Reliability testing and the use of statistics in performance analysis support: a case study from an international netball tournament', in P. G. O'Donoghue and M. Hughes (eds) *Performance Analysis of Sport 6* (pp.1–7), Cardiff: CPA Press, UWIC.

O'Donoghue, P. G. and Robinson, G. (2009) 'Validation of the ProZone3® player tracking system: a preliminary report', *International Journal of Computer Science in Sport*, 8(1): 38–53.

O'Donoghue, P. G. and Williams, J. J. (2004) 'An evaluation of human and computer-based predictions of the 2003 Rugby Union World Cup', *International Journal of Computer Science in Sport*, 3(1): 5–22.

O'Donoghue, P. G., Papadimitriou, K., Gourgoulis, V. and Haralambis, K. (2012) 'Statistical methods in performance analysis: an example from international soccer', *International Journal of Performance Analysis in Sport*, 12: 90–100.

Olsen, E. (1981), *Fotball taktikk*, Oslo: Norwegian School of Sport Sciences.

Perl, J., Tilp, M., Baca, A. and Memmert, D. (2013) 'Neural networks for analysing sports games', in T. McGarry, P. G. O'Donoghue and J. Sampaio (eds) *Routledge handbook of sports performance analysis* (pp. 237–47), London: Routledge.

Prestigiacomo, L. (2003) *Coaching Soccer: Match Strategy and Tactics*, Spring City, PA: Reedswain Publishing.

Punj, G. and Stewart, D. W. (1983) 'Cluster analysis in market research: review and suggestions for application', *Journal of Marketing Research*, 20(2): 134–48.

Rees, C. and James, N. (2006) 'A new approach to evaluating "streakiness" in golf', in H. Dancs, M. D. Hughes and P. G. O'Donoghue (eds) *Performance Analysis of Sport 7* (pp. 352–60) Cardiff: CPA Press.

Robinson, G., O'Donoghue, P. G. and Wooster, B. (2011) 'Path changes in the movement of English Premier League soccer players', *Journal of Sports Medicine and Physical Fitness*, 51(2): 220–6.

252

Robles, F., Castellano, J., Perea, A. and Martínez-Santos, R. (2011) 'Spatial strategy used by the world champions in South Africa 2010', World Congress of Science and Football 7, Book of Abstracts (p. 7), Nagoya, Japan, 26–30 May.

Salkind, N. J. (2004) *Statistics for People Who (Think They) Hate Statistics*, 2nd edn, Thousand Oaks, CA: Sage.

Sarmento, H., Barbosa, A., Anguera, M. T., Campaniço, J. and Leitão, J. (2013) 'Regular patterns of play in the counter-attack of the FC Barcelona and Manchester United football teams', in D. M. Peters and P.G. O'Donoghue (eds) *Performance Analysis of Sport X* (pp. 57–64), London: Routledge.

Shaw, M. J., Subramaniam, C., Tan, G. W. and Welge, M. E. (2001) 'Knowledge management and data mining for marketing', *Decision Support Systems*, 31: 127–37.

Sportstec (2013) SportsCode User Manual, sportscode help files, pp. 162–93.

Szolovits, P. (1982) 'Artificial Intelligence and Medicine', in P. Szolovits (ed), *Artificial Intelligence in Medicine*, Boulder, CO: Westview Press.

Taylor, J. B., Mellalieu, S. D., James, N. and Shearer, U. A. (2008) 'The influence of match location, quality of opposition and match status on technical performance in professional association football', *Journal of Sports Sciences*, 26: 885–95.

Tenga, A. (2010) Reliability and validity of match performance analysis in soccer: a multidimensional qualitative evaluation of opponent interaction, Ph.D. thesis, Norwegian School of Sports Sciences.

Tenga, A., Kanstad, D., Ronglan, L.T. and Bahr, R. (2009) 'Developing a new method for team match performance analysis in professional soccer and testing its reliability', *International Journal of Performance Analysis in Sport*, 9: 8–25.

Tufte, E.R. (2006) *Beautiful Evidence*, Cheshire, CT: Graphics Press.

Vincent, W.J. (1999) *Statistics in Kinesiology*, 2nd edn, Champaign, Il: Human Kinetics Publishers.

Vincent, W.J. and Wier, ?. (2012) *Statistics in Kinesiology*, 4th edn, Champaign, Il: Human Kinetics Publishers.

Wiltshire, H.D. (2013) 'Sports performance analysis for high performance managers', In T. McGarry, P.G. O'Donoghue and J. Sampaio (eds) *Routledge Handbook of Sports Performance Analysis* (pp. 176–86), London: Routledge.

Worthington, E. (1980) *Teaching Soccer Skills*, London: A & C Black Publishers Ltd.

# INDEX

258

Lightning Source UK Ltd.
Milton Keynes UK
UKOW01f1004230915

259128UK00005B/62/P